The
Genesis
of the
Cornwall Air
Ambulance
Service

FROM A DREAM TO REALITY

GEOFF NEWMAN

ISBN: 978-1-4834-7051-1 (sc)
ISBN: 978-1-4834-7052-8 (e)

Because of the dynamic nature of the Internet, any web addresses or links contained in this book may have changed since publication and may no longer be valid. The views expressed in this work are solely those of the author and do not necessarily reflect the views of the publisher, and the publisher hereby disclaims any responsibility for them.

Any people depicted in stock imagery provided by Thinkstock are models, and such images are being used for illustrative purposes only. Certain stock imagery © Thinkstock.

Lulu Publishing Services rev. date: 05/24/2017

Dedication

I would like to dedicate this booklet to the people of Cornwall who kept the Air Ambulance project alive in those critical early years.

ACKNOWLEDGMENTS

My thanks to Paul Westaway for kindly writing the foreword to this booklet. To Milly Knight for help with the cover design and to Nigel Penton Tilbury for help with the images. A special thanks to Paula Martin at the Cornwall Air Ambulance Trust for encouraging me to write this account of the Unit's early history. I hope sales will produce a small but steady contribution to their funds.

FOREWORD

by

Paul Westaway

Senior Paramedic at the start of the Air Ambulance project

As we embarked on a fantastic journey into the unknown Geoff told me, "Paul, this will change your life" … he was absolutely right. Of course, I was not able to fully appreciate the significance of that statement, delivered in a very matter of fact way, at the time; but yes, his prophecy came to pass, and my life has never been the same since we began serving the people of Cornwall on the 1st of April 1987.

It is not only my life that was changed by the Air Ambulance, for countless thousands have benefited from the skill of the crews who fly on the helicopters. They have also benefitted from the sheer speed with which the crews can be delivered to incidents wherever they occur, and when necessary the patients can quickly be flown to an appropriate hospital.

In the period following the launch of the service our long-term future could be counted in just days and weeks. It is, therefore, true to say that none of us, at that time, could have really envisaged the country being served today by over 30 air ambulance helicopters. Some of these are operating 24 hours per day, flying emergency missions on night vision goggles and carrying Doctors along with the latest life-saving equipment.

This tale of how it began features many of the same factors involved at the start of any life-changing project and irreplaceable resource. It invariably includes one person's vision followed by commitment, dedication and absolute single-mindedness. It was this single-mindedness that led to the launch of the Cornwall's Air Ambulance. Geoff Newman and the small but effective group that came together in those early days needed all of these qualities to bring the project to a successful conclusion.

So many events of those early days are brought to life in this book. Geoff records those formative discussions and initial decisions intended to deliver a well-designed operational model. The sheer evangelical zeal that drove the launch of this innovative service still underpins it today and allows the continued delivery of a vital life-saving service.

This is the story that started with one man, who convinced a small but essential team of people that a helicopter Air Ambulance was essential for Cornwall. He was right, not just for Cornwall but the whole of the United Kingdom. The gestation of this project is a very human 'David and Goliath' tale. Here Geoff tells his story. It was an adventure that became, as he says in his own words, 'a life-changing experience'. The Air Ambulance may change your life too one day. To those men and women who listened – we say 'thank you'.

Paul Westaway

INTRODUCTION

I have been asked many times over the last 30 years how did the Air Ambulance in Cornwall begin. Here is my account of how I came across an opportunity and with the help of friends, family and colleagues turned it into a reality.

A project with the impact and profile of the Cornwall Air Ambulance cannot move from concept to successful operation without encountering some hiccups on the way. There are too many egos, committees and problematic aspects of national health service management to be understood and addressed and I certainly had a few hurdles to overcome along the way. However, a window of opportunity, created by an NHS need to address certain shortfalls in the ambulance service at that time, enabled me, with much help from others, to steer events towards a successful conclusion.

That the Cornwall initiative should go on and provide the incentive to others in the UK is a testimony to the successful teamwork of all those involved. This small team created an addition to the ambulance service's capabilities that improved clinical care and acted as a logistical tool that enhanced the overall effectiveness of the land-based service. Perhaps the most appropriate testimony to its success was the creation of a charity by local people that provided the necessary funds to keep it going and was to prove the game-changer for the prospects of the wider use of helicopter air ambulances. I cannot praise the efforts of those involved with fundraising, then and now, enough.

You won't find much, if anything, in the official records about how the ground was prepared before the service contract for the helicopter was signed by the CEO of the Cornwall NHS. It was always a more appropriate PR policy, from the NHS perspective, to present the idea of introducing the air ambulance concept as their own. By allowing the NHS team to drive the PR agenda in this way it was possible for the Head of Primary Care Services (HPCS), to blast and bluster his way through the NHS bureaucracy. It was painful to have all my preparatory work airbrushed from the record in this way, but it was a considered a necessary strategy at the time, and maybe it paid off in the end. It's ironic that it has taken thirty years to put the record straight.

The stresses and strains of that first year of operations took their toll. It followed the six months of virtually unpaid work I put into getting the project to the stage where a contract to provide the service could be signed. Now, 30 years on, I can take perhaps a more measured view of that period. I can appreciate that my commitment and passion for the project may have contributed to the tensions that developed with NHS management. I hope they can understand why I was so passionate about a project that I had taken from the drawing board to a fully functioning air ambulance service.

I am now trying to establish myself as a writer. I have four books self-published to date. Every author needs a good agent and mine is telling me that my role as the man who conceived, designed and established the nation's first air ambulance operation is something I should be proud of. Something I should speak about more so that it brings to people's attention my new role as an author of crime-thriller novels.

I therefore decided to turn a pamphlet, written a few years ago about the genesis of the Air Ambulance, into this more comprehensive booklet packed with interesting facts and photographs along with the relevant pages of my logbook showing details of the first 400+ missions. By using it as a fundraiser, I hope to create a win-win situation that benefits both the Cornwall Air Ambulance Service Trust and my new career as an author.

Geoff Newman
May 2017

WHY DID CORNWALL NEED AN AIR AMBULANCE?

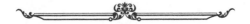

An appropriate place to begin this story may be first to explain why we needed an air ambulance in Cornwall at that time. The Ambulance Service in those days served those living inside the county boundaries. It was funded on a per-capita basis, and while the provisioning formula took into account the influx of millions of tourists, it was by no means generous. It certainly did not consider the difficulties of serving a peninsular with no adjacent counties other than Devon to provide A & E Units close enough to be capable of reducing the delivery time to a hospital. The other problem was that the Ambulance Service was always the 'Prima-Donna' of the NHS finance department. If the Health Authority was short of cash, there was nothing in those days to prevent them raiding the money set aside for the replacement of ambulances and the training of ambulance personnel. The Cornwall Ambulance Service was short of resources in every department and was in need of a 'game-changer'.

The Air Ambulance had the potential to be a tool that could make a real difference – just what Cornwall Ambulance Service needed. Meeting response time targets set by the government was increasingly difficult given that nobody had thought to include in the formula the length of time needed to subsequently deliver a patient to the hospital. In Cornwall, it can take a long time to get to either the one General Hospital in the county, Treliske at Truro, or the equivalent hospital over the border in Devon.

Also, with no allowance for the length of time taken for an ambulance to become available after a call, it was possible for ambulance resources to disappear from the control room map at an alarming rate during busy times of the day.

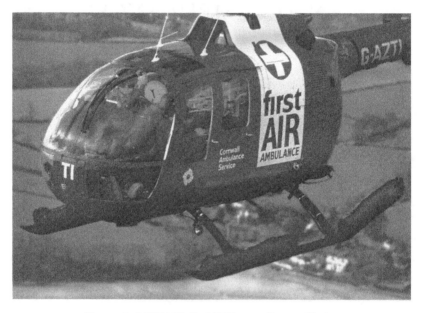

Figure 1- MBB105 G-AZTI over Cornwall 1987

In 1986, the county was served by 17 front line vehicles during daylight and 11 at night. Human activity reduces during the hours of darkness so the same level of service could be provided with fewer resources. The other critical statistic related to the length of the journey to hospital was the time a vehicle took to return to normal service in its nominated operating area. The time taken to answer a call and then 'return to station' is a critical time-span and is one that has enormous implications if your home is in faraway Penzance or Bude.

The technique employed for the location of emergency ambulances at that time had just been changed from basing them in ambulance stations, to spreading them around the county and parking them at strategic locations. The huge map on the control room wall at Truro HQ showed the position of each emergency vehicle and as resources were allocated to the incoming 999 calls so vehicles would be shuffled around the county to optimise the response time for the next call. It was a kind of chess game with the added frisson of nobody knowing when the next move would come nor from where it would come.

If there were an emergency in northeast Cornwall, Bude for example, this would require the emergency ambulance to deliver the patient to Plymouth Freedom Fields Hospital, a journey that would see the vehicle and crew being away from their area for up to four hours.

Another revealing statistic, not collected at the time, was the amount of time the county was without cover altogether. Yes, there were occasions, many actually, when the controllers ran out of resources of available emergency vehicles. That statistic would be a measure of how the resources provided by government correlated with the demand – an altogether inconvenient number. If the Duty Controller were lucky, there would be no calls during that period, and nobody would ever know. But, if not, then they had a serious problem.

The air ambulance could cover virtually the entire county within 20 minutes and help to minimise the impact of these shortcomings. Though not able to land in certain areas, the resourcefulness of the air and ground crews and the ability of this small helicopter to negotiate tiny landing sites or difficult and inaccessible terrain would prove to be a valuable asset when the chips were down. It truly could be a tremendous asset to a service that desperately needed an uplift to its capability.

HOW I CAME TO BE INVOLVED IN THE AIR AMBULANCE PROJECT

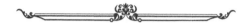

To better understand my attachment to Cornwall perhaps I should explain that in my wife and I have spent most of our married life in the county and at while setting up the air ambulance we were living just outside the village of Perranarworthal.

In the Spring of 1986, I had just returned from China where I had been working as an Aviation Consultant for a consortium of Western oil companies.

The trip had not been particularly successful. It had been organised to support the bid by a British helicopter company to win a contract from the Chinese government to supply a complete Search and Rescue Helicopter Service for the Chinese coastline. We failed to convince them to take up our offer, and we returned to UK empty handed.

The point of this introductory tale is that this was the moment at which I began to research how public helicopter services worked around the world and how our own services might be expanded to include many public service roles such as law enforcement and medical emergencies. As an ex-naval pilot, I knew that the SAR helicopters were capable of much more than just rescuing errant swimmers and fishermen in difficulties. Maybe they could contribute to the needs of ambulance services around the country? They already provided some help and many a difficult spinal injury patient had been delivered to Stoke Mandeville hospital by RAF or Royal Navy helicopter. Unfortunately, I was to find that military resources are not optimised for this kind of service and are fearsomely expensive when compared with the helicopters available in the civilian world.

I looked far and wide to see how other countries organised air ambulances. Eventually, I came upon the German air ambulance system, then the most advanced in Europe. It was established in 1973, and by 1986 there were around twenty air ambulance helicopters serving the German public. Today they have more than fifty air ambulances. My research then took two parallel paths. The first was to try to understand why the UK, an advanced and aviation-oriented country, had failed to introduce an air ambulance system when most European countries either had or were developing, air ambulance services in one form or another. The second was to formulate a strategy that would facilitate the introduction of air ambulances into the UK.

The answer to the first turned out to be quite simple – the way the NHS was organised was the problem or at least the requirement for any initiative for such a service to originate centrally, from the Government in London. The National Health system in the UK is perpetually short of funds, and because it provides a service that is free at the point of delivery, it would always be so. It is funded centrally from government coffers, and the total shared between the hundreds of recipient departments on a 'slice-of-cake' basis. Each department would get its share and only get more if the cake gets bigger or it somehow contrives to 'steal' a portion from someone else's slice.

There is no way the government then, or now for that matter, will commit an organisation like the NHS to a 'big-bucks' item like a national fleet of helicopters that would probably run (today) to more than £100m per year. I was to find out later in the project that the government had been lobbied many times by the company that made the helicopter used by many of the German air ambulance stations. They never really had any prospect of success for when you are faced with a system that is financed using the 'slice of cake' principle, it is virtually impossible to find a section of the NHS willing to sacrifice a portion of their slice of the cake to pay for a newcomer. Only something extraordinary could break the log-jam. I set about searching for a solution.

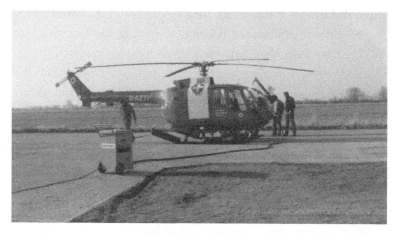

Figure 2 – 'Tango India' is prepared for service in Cornwall at the Cambridgeshire base of Bond Helicopters.

If and when the solution was found I would need to focus on three things, funding, command and control and finally, helicopter selection.

By the early summer of 1986, I was beginning to worry about a shortage of paid work. The helicopter world was a little flat at that time, and both flying and consultancy work was thin on the ground. I was then fortunate to be contacted by two local businessmen who wanted my help in setting up a commercial helicopter operation in the West Country.

My task in this project was to find suitable ways of generating commercial charter business. I was also tasked with managing the technicalities relating to obtaining an operating licence from the Civil Aviation Authority. Our relationship began very positively, and I was optimistic that something might come of our deliberations.

During my research into the way our emergency services operated I came across The National Health Service Year Book, a reference book that covered every area of the NHS. With its help, I was able to sketch out the boundaries of the various Health Authorities and establish who was the responsible person in each department. If I were ever to engage with the NHS, then this 'bible' would be my guide to who to contact and where they could be found.

At the time, I was also researching the way the German Air Ambulance system was organised and discovered something quite remarkable. Most missions they conducted did NOT require the transportation of the patient. Their experience was that in most cases the medical crew were able to stabilise and treat the patient at the scene and only in a few extreme cases was it necessary to use the helicopter to transport the patient. The remainder of the time the normal road ambulance would carry the patient if transportation was required after stabilisation.

This simple fact was critical for then it was possible to imagine a regular charter helicopter being used to deliver the medical crew and their portable equipment to the scene of an incident. By describing a helicopter as 'normal' what I mean is the kind of helicopter that the two businessmen envisage purchasing for their enterprise. A Bell JetRanger or an AS350 Squirrel.

For those that are unfamiliar with the implications of this, I should explain that an executive charter helicopter is expensive enough, but the costs of converting one to carry a stretcher patient and all the bespoke equipment needed to monitor and support the patient adds hugely to the total. Worse than that, a medically equipped helicopter cannot easily be used for any other type of work so the income stream needed to support a medical helicopter would have to be substantial for it would have to be a dedicated resource. Back in 1986 a suitable second-hand helicopter would probably have cost in the region of £500,000 and fitting it out for the air ambulance role would add another £100,000 to £200,000. Avoiding those additional expenses would make the whole project more viable.

I talked through the concept of using their machine to deliver the medical crew with the businessmen, and they were enthusiastic. The idea had caught their imagination. Unfortunately, the project stalled while we tried to find a way of financing a trial of the 'one-way' air ambulance concept. Not long after, I came across an article in Flight International magazine about the commercial sponsorship by a bank of a 'Surf Rescue' helicopter in Australia. I thought I had discovered the golden key to success and immediately began researching how charities obtained commercial sponsorship in the UK. Could we find enough money through sponsorship to pay the bills? Some homework would clearly be required, and we all realised that the best way to convince a sponsor that the idea was viable would be to start the operation ourselves - provided we could find the money. The businessmen said they thought it was possible and they set to work with the people that controlled their extensive financial resources.

To give the task of raising funds for the air ambulance some perspective, I looked into how the RNLI was funded. I discovered that they raised money in many different ways and the previous year (1985) had seen £24m deposited in tins, raffles, plastic lifeboats and many other clever ideas designed to tug at the heartstrings - and purse strings - of sailors and non-sailors alike. That kind of money would fund a nationwide network of air ambulances and while the RNLI might save 1500 lives, each year air ambulances could make a significant contribution to the saving of twice that number. If they could do it maybe, we could too. Perhaps we could add charitable funds to our list of possible financial supporters.

On the command and control side, I was trying to understand what sort of creature the monolithic NHS was. This is a little like wandering around a huge beached whale trying to find the correct orifice through which an intelligent conversation may be had. Understanding the complexities of the NHS is a huge challenge for the uninitiated.

I did discover that the law in the UK specifically made the provision of emergency response ambulances the responsibility of the Health Authority (now Health Trusts). Previous attempts by diverse organisations that included the Devon and Cornwall Police in partnership with the Devon and Exeter Accident and Emergency Unit had failed to operate as well as they could have done because they thought they could go over the heads of the Ambulance Service. Unfortunately, the odds were stacked against them. The only way forward was to work with the Ambulance Service.

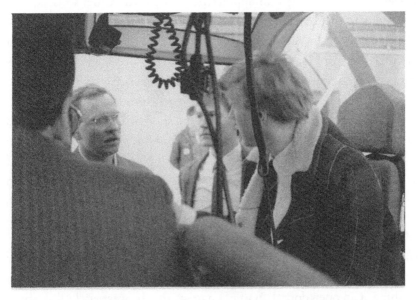

Figure 3 – A&E Consultant Nigel Selwood and Senior Paramedic Paul Westaway discuss the clinical issues during the visit to Germany in early 1987

By Summer I was idly considering the siting of a commercial helicopter able to do part-time Air Ambulance work at either Gloucester Airport or Exeter Airport and shared my thoughts with the businessmen. They were intrigued and wanted me to pursue the project further.

The turning point was the day I discovered from my NHS 'bible' that there were five separate ambulance services serving the territory within the target 20-minute flight time from Gloucester Airport. Knowing, as I do, the kind of turf wars that neighbouring state organisations contrive to indulge in I decided to think again. The prospect of getting five different ambulance services to agree on a common way forward would be nothing short of impossible, at least in any sensible timescale. My wife Lesley came up with the idea of contacting our local Ambulance Service in Truro.

It wasn't difficult to get an appointment to see the Chief Officer, Len Holden, and the following day I walked into his office at the Ambulance HQ in Truro. On the wall behind Len's desk was a large poster of a German Air Ambulance Helicopter. I knew immediately that this was going to be an important day for the project. Len was very patient, and he listened to all my ideas about how we could get commercial sponsorship to pay for a German style service. I asked question after question about his organisation and how it was put together and how it was organised. He was very helpful then he asked me where I was planning such a venture. I said 'Gloucester'. He shrugged his shoulders and said, 'why don't you do it here, in Cornwall?'

My chin must have smacked on my chest with those words. It was the first time I had encountered a positive attitude about the idea of an air ambulance within the NHS, and it seemed that I might, for once, be pushing at an open door. Len went on to say that he was very bullish about starting a helicopter project in Cornwall because he now had a new Head of Primary Care Services (HPCS) and a new and progressive Accident and Emergency consultant, Nigel Selwood, supervising his operation.

He kindly organised a meeting with his boss, The Head of Primary Care Services (HPCS), at his St Austell office.

At that meeting, I learnt that the Health Authority had discussed the use of a helicopter to assist with long distance transfers to Bristol and London, but they had never considered the benefits of an air ambulance that worked as a 'front-line' unit in the way that the German model did.

Len was a vital link in the chain of events that led to our ultimate success, and for that, we owe him a lot. The fact that the HPCS was a retired aviator would mean that we spoke the same language even if his 'dialect' turned out to be the fixed wing variety.

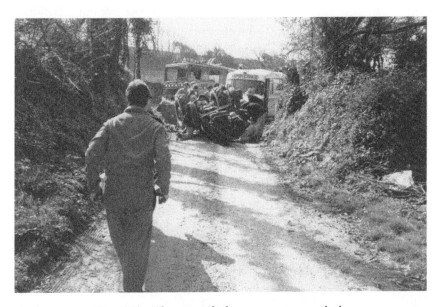

Figure 4 - The air ambulance crew approach the scene of a road accident. The driver was pinned by the legs under his upturned tractor

Such was the degree of enthusiasm for the concept of a full-service medical helicopter coming from both the businessmen and the HPCS that the 'one-way' version faded in favour of going the whole hog and setting up a dedicated helicopter unit. It was agreed that the best hope for raising the necessary finance would come from commercial sponsorship. It was agreed that the businessmen would provide the initial finance to get the project under way. Unfortunately, as things turned out, there was a chicken and egg situation. They were unlikely to be able to get access to the necessary funds without knowing for sure where the income to pay the bills would eventually come from.

I took the news of my meeting with the HPCS to the businessmen in about August of '86. On the back of their confidence, we put a business plan together, arranged for the businessmen to visit Germany with me to see the German Helicopter Emergency Medical Service (HEMS) at work.

When we returned, we started looking around for a suitable helicopter and were able to locate some second-hand MBB105s that were being sold by one of the UK's leading helicopter operators – Bond Helicopters, a family run firm specialising in the offshore oil market. I had previously worked for Bond as a North Sea helicopter pilot and held them in high regard.

By the beginning of September, we had a preliminary plan we could put before the Health Authority. The HPCS had charted a possible course through the minefields of Health Authority committees. The man was a consummate politician and excellent public speaker.

During the first week of September, I had the summons to attend a meeting with the businessmen. There I was briefed on the progress to date. The most important points included being told that I was expected to train the younger businessman to Commercial Pilot's Licence standard (he had a helicopter Private Pilot's License) on the (to-be-acquired) helicopter so that he could be a member of the air ambulance crew. The structure of the new company was explained, and it was clear that despite having an obvious training role I did not, otherwise, feature in their plans for the new company.

'What would be my position in the company?' I asked,

'You don't have one,' was the reply.

'What the......... why,' I said.

'Our advice, Geoff, is that because you are not able to invest any cash in this project you are not entitled to any shares, therefore, no directorship or any other formal position in the Company'.

I remember leaving with my emotions aglow. I didn't know what to feel, angry or disappointed. I settled for disappointed. Not only did they want me to do the impossible – train one businessman to CPL standard in less than three months - but they expected this newly qualified pilot with no commercial experience, to fly air ambulance missions that are amongst the most demanding in the helicopter world. It was ridiculous, and the fact that they didn't realise that it was ridiculous meant that I was dealing with a couple of guys who had no real idea about the hugely challenging task that lay ahead. All this without receiving a position or stake in the company in return for all the effort I had put into the project up to that point!

I stopped on the way home and explained on the phone what had happened to my wife. I had worked, unpaid, for months on this project and all my efforts appeared to have foundered. We arranged to meet in Truro and sat in Bustopher Jones's restaurant working out what to do next.

We decided to approach a Financial Advisor friend of ours to try to raise enough money to buy the helicopter. The analysts didn't like my business plan, so I resolved to do it the only other way possible. Take the project to a reputable helicopter company. This, in fact, was a better idea and would ensure that this unique opportunity had the very best chance of success.

The next day I called Stephen Bond, the head of Bond Helicopters, at his office at Bourn near Cambridge. I'm pretty sure that he had been keeping an eye on what we were up to ever since we appeared at his hangar to inspect the elderly MBB105 helicopters that he was selling off. When I spoke to him, I said…

"Stephen, my name is Geoff Newman, I've been working on a project that I think you will be interested in. Can I come and talk to you about it?"

"Sure," he said.

So, on Saturday, September 13th, my 17th wedding anniversary, I drove to Bourn. The meeting was very positive, and Stephen said he would get back to me.

He came back the following week with the message that he wanted to be involved'.

"What do you need to make the most of this opportunity?" he asked.

"I need one of your MBB105s. fitted out for the Air Ambulance role, free of monthly lease charges for three months."

"Crikey Geoff! You don't want much, do you?"

"Stephen", I replied, "if you give me that helicopter virtually free of charge then nobody in the Health Authority management will be able to resist our proposal. All we need is the ability to show what we can do and, if what happens in other parts of Europe can be used as a guide, we will have a very large foot in the door".

If there is one family to whom we in Cornwall, and the rest of the country for that matter, should be grateful, it is Stephen Bond and his three brothers, Geoff, Mike and Peter. If the original idea was mine and the political clout was clearly with our Head of Primary Care Services, then it was Stephen's vision and commitment (and money) that eventually led to a nationwide network of air ambulances. His motives may not have been entirely altruistic (his company now has a significant part of the air ambulance business in the UK), but without his contribution, at a critical time, we would almost certainly be a long way from where we are today.

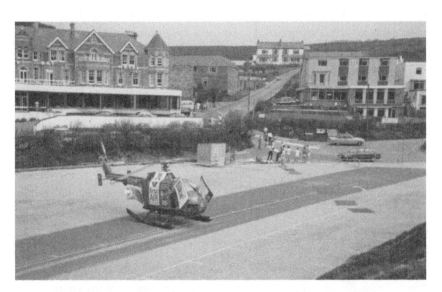

Figure 5 – Attending an injured cyclist at Watergate Bay

I never saw nor heard from the two businessmen again although I understand that they eventually went on to set up their helicopter company. I can imagine that they continued to have a dialogue with the HPCS, but if they did, he never mentioned it to me. I often wonder if they had any regrets about the way they handled things or whether they realise now that the air ambulance project was well beyond their capabilities at that time. I would like to think that they are proud of the small but important part played during the gestation of the air ambulance project. They provided the incentive for me to push on with the idea, and who knows, maybe Stephen Bond thought that if he did not seize the opportunity then maybe the newcomers would.

We went through a period of familiarising the Bond team with the NHS managers in Cornwall, but once they had made each other's acquaintance, everything seemed to come to a grinding halt. By the end of October, I was frustrated by the lack of progress, so I decided to jigger things along a bit. Some years previously I had been asked to do an evaluation on a helicopter service contract that involved Bond Helicopters as one of the bidders. In my files, I had a copy of their standard offshore service contract. Reading this through carefully, I realised that it could be modified to suit the air ambulance task we had envisaged. I set to work and changed it. The suitably modified contract was then put before both Bond and the NHS and with something to chew on the ball was once again rolling. The Health Authority now had something definite to put in front of the various committees, and they got to work.

By December 1986 we were able to stage a formal contract signing at the Bassett Count House restaurant near Redruth. The HPCS was concerned that the news of the deal would cause some problems amongst the unions within the Ambulance Service. He, therefore, ordered total secrecy and then extraordinarily announced that despite the contract instructions to the contrary, he would take over the raising of commercial sponsorship. Fundraising was supposed to be my responsibility as the nominal Project Manager. I had all the contacts lined up to take the process forward, but the HPCS recognised that with Bond Helicopters committed to the project he now had the whip hand and demanded total control of every aspect. It was necessary to 'wind my neck in' and keep my fingers crossed that he would deliver the goods.

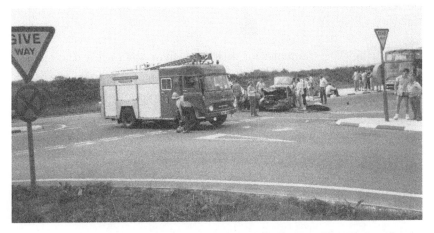

Figure 6 - This road accident occurred at Goss Moor and required the attendance of the Fire and Rescue Service to extract the occupants from their seriously damaged vehicle

The following months were agony. We had so much to do and couldn't breathe a word about it. The start date was fixed for April 1st, 1987 to commemorate the day the RAF was born.

The term 'paramedic' was not in the official NHS lexicon at this time, but many of the skills associated with their role were available to some Ambulance Technicians who were then designated 'Extended Trained'. All our Technicians were in this category which was then a new and scarce resource.

Paul Westaway was to be the group trainer and had responsibility for designing the modus-operandi for the ambulance guys. I had the task of preparing the paramedics for their new role as well as designing the operating system for the dispatch and deployment of the helicopter. We could not use the German model for they always carried a Trauma Doctor. We would have to make it work with two paramedics. We would also have to operate within the constraints of the Public Transport Regulations with very few 'easements'.

In preparing the paramedics for their new environment, I had to include some aspects of what would usually be considered to be the copilot's duties. With no autopilot to 'fly' the helicopter, I was constantly 'hands-on'. At best, I could apply some friction on the collective lever so that I could free my left hand to operate switches and tune radios. My medical colleagues would have to help with the navigation and read out the pre-take-off and pre-landing checklists. They would also have to learn about the relevant safety procedures and how to manage the landing site after our arrival. It was always necessary to run the engines (and rotors) for two minutes after landing to cool vital parts of the turbine before stopping them. Making the area around the helicopter safe for people to walk around was an essential part of our safety procedures. The crew would have to protect the helicopter during this period.

The first guys were: Paul Westaway i/c, Bob Alderson, Chris Prissell, Nigel Harris, Mark O'Byrne, Simon Williams, Les Slade & David Triggs. The training course I devised and delivered for the paramedics was a week long and covered everything from basic mathematics and geometry to Air Law and navigation. We also introduced them to the naval tradition called 'Wet Dinghy Drill'. We had some fun; they were enthusiastic students.

My position as a contract pilot with Bond had been confirmed back in December when, if I recollect correctly, they put me on half pay. Come April 1st that would go up to full pay and would equate to the typical scale for a Bond Captain on the MBB105. It was the lowest pay grade in the company, but beggars can't be choosers. It was good to be on the receiving end of a regular income for a change.

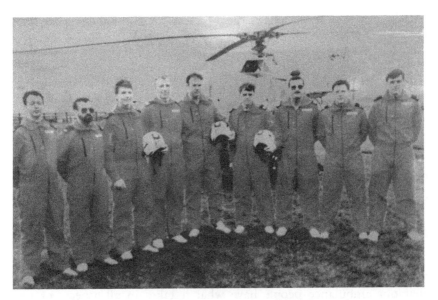

Figure 7- L to R - Nigel, Les, Paul, Chris,
Self, Bob, Mark, Simon, Dave

My schedule included a six-week period working in the Operations Room learning everything there was to learn about how the Ambulance Service marshalled and deployed its resources. The patterns of the ambulance service activity were studied and studied until we realised that there was only one basic pattern. The higher the level of human activity the higher the rate of emergency calls. We used this simple fact to guide our selection of working times and working days. I was scheduled to be the only pilot on the project until there was enough cash to pay for another. That meant that we could only work for 10 hours a day, five days a week. We had to work out which days and what hours to cover.

The clinical management of the Ambulance Service was down to their A & E consultant, the newly arrived Dr Nigel Selwood. It was our good fortune that Nigel was very receptive to our project and his support and clinical direction ensured that the crews were in the best possible shape to deliver a much more sophisticated level of pre-hospital care than had been possible before.

While discussions were going on D-Day was approaching. I went out on the road in a front-line ambulance to experience the adrenalin rush that comes with a 'red call'. If there is one group of guys and girls that are grossly undervalued in our community, it's the ambulance men and women. These days most are paramedic qualified and play a vital role in our society. The TLC that they deliver in difficult... wrong! .... tough circumstances have to be seen to be believed.

I experienced for the first time the strength that a seriously ill patient with a heart attack gets just by holding your hand. Bodily contact is not something we Anglo-Saxons are very good at, but we can feel confident that our ambulance people have what it takes in all aspects of the professional skills required to do the job.

With a month or so to go, I confessed to Paul that I was concerned about the problems with dealing with all the blood and gore at the scene of a bad accident and what would he advise.

He recommended a short visit to the morgue. He took me along to observe proceedings and then disappeared, returning 4 hours later. In the meantime, the mortuary assistants gave me lessons on the conduct of post-mortems. They made use of my presence by asking me to assist with the collection and weighing of organs. It was certainly a unique and valuable experience, but I didn't sleep properly for three days afterwards. It seemed to do the trick. Funny how your mind can compensate when you have tough stuff to do. That reminds me, I still owe Paul for pulling that trick on me.

D-Day was almost upon us, and we had to come to terms with the fact that the HPCS's strategy for raising commercial sponsorship had not been a success. We had just enough funding for 90 days and would have to show we could perform pretty quickly.

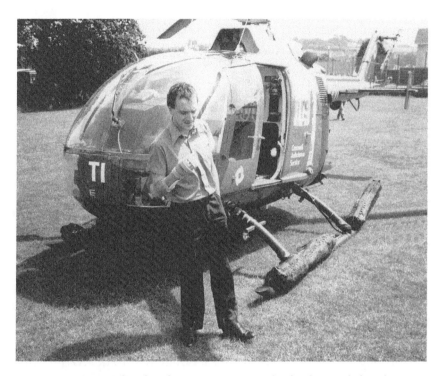

Figure 8 - This chap became a customer the day he tangled with a huge circular saw at his workplace. He suffered a traumatic amputation of his right hand but due to the prompt actions of his colleagues and the skill of the surgeons it was reattached later that day. He saw us landing at an incident and came over to thank us and to have his picture taken with Tango India. Rapid transportation to definitive care was the key.

In the run-up to the start date, we arranged a visit to Germany. The Head of Primary Care, the A&E Consultant, the Chief Ambulance Officer and Paul Westaway came along to see how the medical crew functioned and what equipment they used. It was a significant opportunity for those unfamiliar with the difficulties of managing a patient when you are in the air. Nigel, the A&E consultant, had brought along a list of clinical conditions that he planned to exclude from our mission capabilities. He was amazed to hear from the leading expert in Munich that this was completely the wrong approach.

"You cannot tell somebody who is having a heart attack on a mountainside that you don't want him to fly because flying might be stressful. You must do your best to save him and deliver him to definitive care. To do less would condemn the man to die. No, you must only exclude from the helicopter those patients that represent a danger to the machine and its crew. If they are combative and you have doubts about being able to restrain them then do not fly them."

Our consultant came away very impressed and greatly reassured about what could and what could not be done in the confines of a small helicopter.

While I was busy doing my research at Ambulance HQ in Cornwall during the early months of 1987 a team of engineers at the Bond Helicopters HQ was carrying out the necessary modifications to MBB105 G-AZTI. This machine was already 'elderly' by the time I arrived at Bourn to test fly it, but it had been thoroughly overhauled and sported a new coat of paint, and a new livery would soon proclaim its status in the UK. Stephen Bond's advertising agency had come up with a title for the unit that went straight to the heart of the issue. 'FIRST AIR AMBULANCE' was born.

We would be the first air ambulance helicopter unit in the UK to operate as a front-line unit capable of independently delivering an emergency response capability. This fact was not lost on the Bond management and certainly not on the UK Civil Aviation Authority. The Bond Chief Pilot had to be sure that we would be able to deliver a safe operation regardless of its effectiveness. This would be the first time that a civilian, non-SAR helicopter unit, working under the strict regulations that govern commercial aviation, would attempt to respond to a call for assistance without knowing exactly where it would be landing. The concept was simple, but the execution was fraught with danger. One serious incident or God forbid, an accident, and it would probably be our last. In the USA, this type of helicopter service is found in every State but during the five years running up to the start of our service there had been so many fatal accidents in America that the whole concept was being called into question. I was confident, however, that a well-trained and disciplined unit could deliver a safe service. I had to show that we were prepared, so I organised some dummy training missions to prove our command and control system and to validate our crew concept.

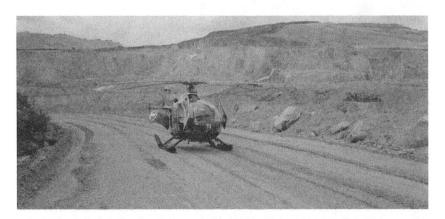

Figure 9 - Attending an incident in the Clay Pits near St Austell

We planned on a normal crew of three, pilot plus two paramedics. When we set off on a mission, the paramedic in the 'co-pilot' seat faces forward to assist with the navigation. When a patient is carried, the copilot's seat is reversed so that the paramedic can manage the patient's airway. It is usually my job to remove the quick-release fittings and turn the seat around, but all crew members had to be able to do it correctly so that would be part of our training too. None of the paramedics had ever flown in a helicopter before, so each was given the opportunity to fly in the front seat and the rear, side-facing seat. I think most suffered from nerves but put a brave face on things. All were excited about the challenge ahead. It wasn't going to be easy, but we were all determined to make it work.

One of the training missions was to a simulated patient inside on the first floor of a farmhouse just outside Helston. This mission had been arranged with Hayden Wallis a local farmer and fellow Rotarian. He had the privilege of being the first 'civilian' to be loaded into 'Tango India'. All of the equipment carried in the helicopter was new, and most of it was 'state-of-the-art' and had been begged or borrowed from the manufacturers or their distributors. The essentials were carried in specially made backpacks that enabled the crew to transport them to the accident or incident scene if the helicopter was unable to land nearby.

During the pre-start-up phase, we had decided to develop a unique modus operandi to make the most of our capabilities. Our contribution was designed to add to the quality of service in two ways. The first was a clinical facet of the service and the second a logistical one.

The fact that we had ambulance personnel trained to paramedic standard was a huge improvement in the quality and quantity of therapies available at the scene of an accident or medical incidents such as a stroke or heart attack. The reader must remember that in 1987 we were still running an ambulance service in which the crews wore blue serge suits and were trained to deliver 'first aid'. They had access to oxygen therapy, Entonox pain control therapy and some had begun to learn how to provide infusion therapy. To this, the paramedic could add a variety of drug therapies and the ability to intubate patients when necessary.

He was also trained to use a defibrillator-heart monitor and had access to other enhanced monitoring equipment that is commonplace today – the Oxygen Sensor and the Blood Pressure monitor - but back then these had to be begged or borrowed for they were very expensive and not available as battery powered self-contained units. Monitoring a critically ill patient is vital, but this is tough inside a noisy helicopter without this specialised equipment.

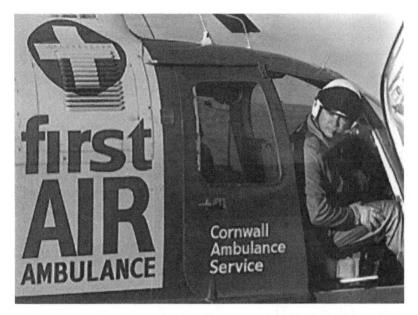

Figure 10 Geoff at the helm of Tango India

The paramedic represented a quantum leap forward in the quality of care available throughout the county. The helicopter would ensure that this limited resource would be available to the entire population of Cornwall and The Isles of Scilly.

The logistical dilemma was one that was essentially a speed and distance problem. The faster a patient can be delivered to definitive care the sooner the ambulance resources are available for the next call. For the road vehicles in the outer edges of the county, this was a serious issue. If you lived in West Penwith, The Lizard or northeast Cornwall then it was a very big problem. For the rest of us, there was a knock-on effect on the response time. It must be remembered that when an ambulance vacates its operating area, the adjacent vehicle is moved to cover that area as well as its original one. That would mean a longer journey for the next call no matter what.

Our intention was to tackle this speed and distance equation in two ways. The first involved the creation of a network of good quality landing areas in strategic locations around the county. These would be used as 'rendezvous' sites so that the ambulance could use the nearest landing area to meet with the helicopter and transfer the patient to the hospital using the air ambulance. The emergency ambulance then remained in its operating area, and the patient was delivered to the hospital in minutes rather than hours. This offered a huge benefit because the first call may be something comparatively minor whereas the second call could be a life-saver. Had the ambulance set off on the long journey to Truro or Plymouth then it would have missed the more urgent call.

A friend of a friend kindly arranged for me to use his light aircraft to reconnoitre these 'secondary' landing sites. One sunny day we flew all around the county and took pictures of areas we thought would be suitable and then set off by car to check out the shortlist.

This technique was to prove to be a fantastic tool in the ambulance service's 'toolbox' during the August Bank Holiday when the roads became so choked that the whole of the west country was completely jammed up from Penzance to Exeter. The emergency ambulance in Camelford had already delivered its patient to Truro, but the Police advised that there was no chance of it getting back to its station. Another 999 call came in from the Camelford area, and the Wadebridge vehicle was mobilised but once on the way to Plymouth there would be just one emergency ambulance in Bude to cover the whole of the northeast of the county.

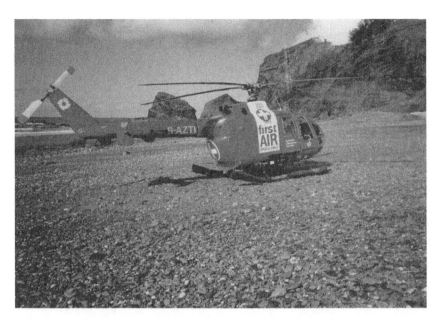

*Figure 11 - Attending to incidents on the county's beaches
was a frequent requirement but only if they were above
the high-water mark. Below that was the responsibility
of the naval Search and Rescue unit at RNAS*

During the months of preparation for the start of the service, I had spent many hours talking with the Ops Room Manager. We had agreed that we would try to keep an open mind about which tasks we could manage and which would be beyond our capabilities; I told him, if in doubt, just ask. On this occasion, he called me with an imaginative and extraordinary request. There was a spare ambulance at Camelford Ambulance Station but no crew. Would we be able to fly the crew stranded in Truro to our regular landing site for the area – Davidstow Moor disused airfield? I discussed the situation with the crew and did some calculations. We had the ability to carry two stretcher patients, but normally our backpacks were stowed on the right-hand stretcher. By moving those to the rear loading area, we would be able to carry both the ambulance men, one on each stretcher. The two guys were a little apprehensive, but both went along with the plan and enjoyed the somewhat unorthodox flight. We christened this our 'Business Class' service.

We arranged to meet the Wadebridge vehicle and take their patient on to Plymouth, leaving them to take the other crew to Camelford to pick up their new ambulance. Within the hour, we had a situation where instead of having just one vehicle in the whole of northeast Cornwall there were now three. From that day on, we carried a set of keys for every ambulance station in the county.

As things turned out it was just as well for that day we completed that first mission and were then tasked to Tintagel – not once – but over the next four hours we were sent to Tintagel for three more emergencies. Our innovative master plan had saved the day in a most unusual way. The local vehicle answered the call, and we transported the patient – perfect!

The second way we wanted to tackle the logistical problems was to use the air ambulance to answer both 999 emergency calls and the so-called 'Urgent' calls. The former are often much less critical than they may at first appear to the unqualified member of the public making the 999 call whereas the latter were guaranteed to be critical but because 'Urgent' calls were initiated by a GP. These could be allocated a notional response time that was longer than the 'immediate' response to a 999 call. In future, any 'Urgent call that presented a logistical problem for the controllers could be considered for the air ambulance when resources were getting low.

This was to prove a contentious issue for the Air Ambulance project wasn't supported by all, and the detractors made the most of every flight that appeared to be for something minor, and that could not justify the use of an expensive resource. I am sad to say that to avoid bad publicity the old attitude of 'can-do' was replaced by a more cautious and arguably more pragmatic policy of avoiding such missions where possible. It is a shame that the true capabilities of the service have not been realised and have been sacrificed on the altar of 'good publicity' or rather, avoiding the chance of bad publicity.

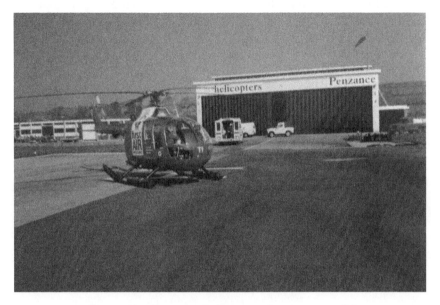

Figure 12 - Penzance heliport was to prove a useful place to transfer patients and for refuels

When resources are stretched, the controllers have to prioritise, and of course, the life-threatening situations have ultimate priority. One day we were told that a lady waiting to go into a hospice was standing at the end of her remote country lane waiting to be picked up by the ambulance. She had been waiting for an hour, but there was no prospect of getting a vehicle to her for the next three hours. There was every prospect of her standing at the end of her lane for all that time with no way to contact her, so we were asked to take on the job. In the normal scheme of things, you could not imagine a more inappropriate way to use an air ambulance but for that elderly lady, on that day, in those circumstances, we were able to deliver a service for which she was very grateful.

It is a pity that, in my opinion, we don't look at the service as a whole rather than try to deploy the air ambulance using a formula designed to protect it from criticism by people who don't understand the big picture. Every 999 call in those days required the mandatory attendance of an emergency ambulance, so a valuable resource was often wasted on patients that did not require it. These days, of course, we have the benefit of paramedics on motorbikes and in rapid response vehicles as well as being allowed to triage the 999 calls so maybe the problems are not quite the same, maybe. There was a third type of mission that we were occasionally asked to perform, and that was the inter-hospital transfer. There are specialist centres for specific types of injury, and sometimes we had to take patients who had spinal injuries or burns to these national or regional centres of excellence. To summarise then, we were faced with three different types of mission:

Primary – The helicopter responds directly to the scene of the incident or accident, and the pilot selects a suitable landing site using his experience and judgement.

Secondary – The helicopter responds to a pre-surveyed landing site, collects a patient from an emergency ambulance and delivers the patient to the hospital. The emergency ambulance is then able to return to its designated operating area to await the next 999 call.

Tertiary – Inter-hospital - transfers patient to a specialist centre.

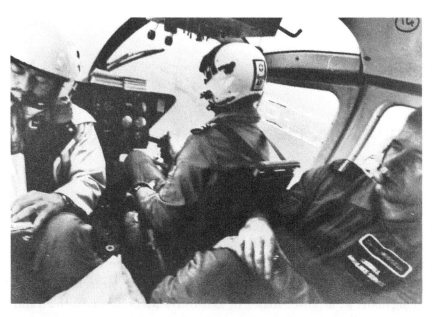

Figure 13 - The MBB105 is a very 'cosy' place in which to work. Here Nigel is busy with the paperwork whilst Chris looks after the patient. We could only afford two crew helmets and poor Chris was the only one they did not fit.

THE END OF THE BEGINNING

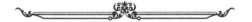

The launch day came, and despite our best efforts the first mission allocated to the helicopter turned out to be inappropriate and not in an appropriate location. To minimise the embarrassment and save on flying hours we deployed to nearby Davidstow Moor disused airfield and awaited developments. As you can imagine, I was not enjoying this first mission one iota. We were all tense and expectant and were desperate for a successful first day.

It wasn't long before we received a call to Porthcurno where a young female student had received a spinal injury while rock climbing. There was a road crew on scene, and they had requested assistance for not only was the patient a long way from the location of the ambulance across a mile of sandy beach but the nature of her injury required the most careful handling. A long carry and then a bumpy ride in a road vehicle was not going to be the best way of taking her to the hospital. The mission went well, and the young lady became famous as the first patient to be transported by the nation's first air ambulance helicopter.

There is a memorable tale that arose from the delivery of that first patient to the safety of Treliske Hospital. She looked up at our paramedic, Nigel Harris, as she was unloaded from the helicopter and said, "This is a wonderful service you have here in Cornwall, how long have you been running?" Nigel looked at his watch and replied, "Since about eight thirty this morning actually."

Once we had completed the first day and with the tension eased, we settled into the routine of answering the daily string of emergencies that came our way. We had elected not to preclude any call from our 'can-do' list. We took everything that came our way and had some remarkable days. When I read through my pilot's logbook today, I can recall in almost every detail some extraordinary emergency calls and the occasional trawl through my box of old photographs brings back poignant memories. I thought the reader would also find these details interesting so at the back of this booklet, you will find a transcription of pages 7 to 30 from Volume Three of my Pilot's Log. I've also included some photographs taken during these missions. When you read through them, you will be perusing the details of the first 400 plus missions flown by a helicopter air ambulance in the UK.

NOTABLE MISSIONS

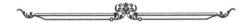

As you read through the fascinating list of missions we undertook during that first year you will marvel at the variety. We saw extremes almost every day. Death and destruction on the roads, death and despair at homes. Tragedy in a country cottage, sadness in a council terrace, joy in a child surviving a disaster, relief at our arrival. Happiness was a noisy red blob that arrives out of nowhere and delivered skilled care and compassion.

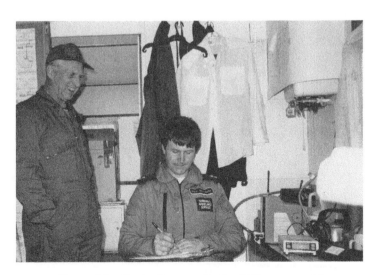

Figure 14 – Senior Paramedic Paul Westaway with our maintenance engineer Peter Rhodes

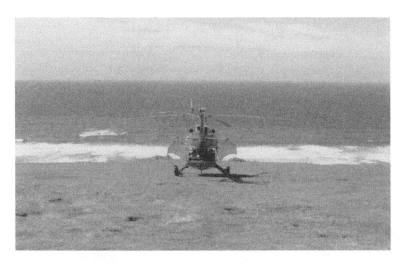

Figure 15 - This iconic picture of Tango India was taken on the cliff-tops north of Newquay. A hang glider 'pilot' had crashed nearby and needed some assistance.

The saving of life in this business is all a question of teamwork. To survive the worst a chain of events must occur that requires everyone from the first responder to the surgeon to do their bit. In that respect, we helped to save quite a few lives by making our contribution. There was one occasion, however when we can honestly say that we were the critical element in the sequence of events that day. It happened on September 26th, 1987. A young teenage lad was riding his trail bike around the cliffs and beaches of the Scillies when he came a cropper and smacked his head on a rock.

The ambulance driver that came to pick him up was apparently his dad. It must have been a shock. The lad wasn't wearing a helmet, so the injury to his skull was severe. The doctor at the hospital on St Mary's immediately recognised the signs of a bleed inside the skull that was pressurising the brain. He called for the air ambulance and arranged for his patient to be flown directly to Freedom Fields Hospital in Plymouth. We arrived, collected the lad and his mother and took them to the landing site in the

Freedom Fields Park. He was rushed into the scanner while the surgical team stood by. We were told that as he came out of the scanner, he died but was then resuscitated. The operation took place immediately, and two days later he was sitting up in bed chatting with his mum when one of our team stopped by to say hello. The flight to the Scilly Isles and back to Plymouth took just one hour and forty minutes.

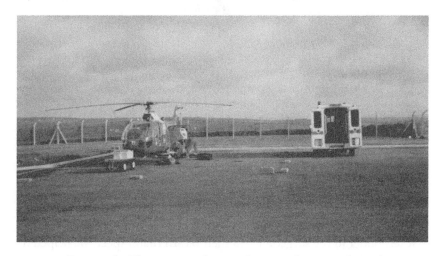

Figure 16 - The compound we used as a parking area housed our fuel bowser (provided for us by BP) our battery cart (used for starting) and our standby ambulance (used for transferring patients down to A & E and when we were grounded by bad weather).

We received tremendous support from the majority of the press, but there was a hard-core of opposition that remained active and vocal throughout. The news reporters local and national would come to see us in our sparse accommodation up at the car park outside CSSD, the NHS Sterilisation Unit at Treliske Hospital. My wife and I were very fortunate to meet Jill Dando who came to our cottage and interviewed us for Spotlight South West. Such a charming young woman. What a tragedy that she should die in such a ghastly way.

Our operating base was inside a compound that belonged to the Hospital Sterilising Centre. We lived in a tiny and ancient caravan that had once seen service as a mobile screening unit. There were tea making facilities, a telephone, a fax and that was about it. The helicopter was parked inside the fenced car parking compound and protected overnight by a tailor-made cover. Our engineer was a tremendous guy called Peter Rhodes. Peter was semi-retired and lived a few miles away. He had accumulated a wealth of experience looking after helicopters all over the world and was a very competent and conscientious member of our team.

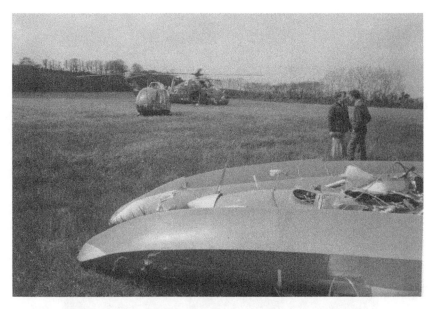

Figure 17 - Tango India and Culdrose SAR meet at the scene of an air crash. A replica of the Schneider Trophy float plane crashed onshore at Mylor Harbour killing the pilot.

Sometime after we began operations, a chap who sold 'T' Shirts offered to make a special version for us that could be sold as a fundraiser so we began the process of raising money with a view to putting it aside ready for the day when someone would have to pay for the service. The 'T' Shirts sold well and later we were asked to sell 'First Air Bears' – Teddy Bears with a shirt sporting the 'First Air' logo. BP Oils had agreed to supply us with a fuel bowser, and I believe the fuel was also supplied free of charge at that time.

Cash was trickling in, but that kind of fund-raising would never be enough. The three-month trial was extended and then extended again. Eventually, a charity based in Camelford was set up and took over financing the helicopter. That part of the story is for others to tell.

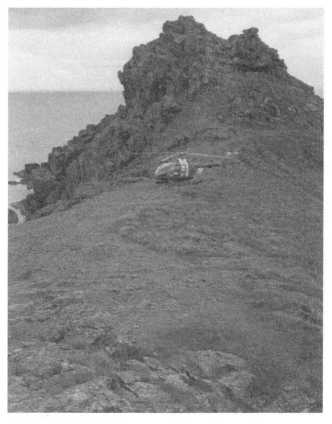

Figure 18 - The coastal footpath was a popular venue for broken limbs.

We knew we had a winner but the battle to keep the unit flying created enormous stresses and strains and the tensions within our group were also beginning to take their toll. By the end of the year, I was ready for a change. I wasn't sleeping, and I was beginning to show the signs of long term fatigue. I knew that if I carried on having to bear the pressure to succeed it could lead to me making errors and that may endanger my colleagues and the future of the operation. Stephen Bond was very understanding but was disappointed by my decision to leave. I think that despite his concern he could see that it was the best all round solution.

I would hand over to Stephen's brother, Geoff Bond. Geoff had taken over in the summer for a couple of weeks so that I could have a break so I knew my paramedic colleagues would be in safe hands. I was asked to stay on and work in the unit servicing the nation's lighthouses, but I knew in my heart of hearts that I needed a complete change.

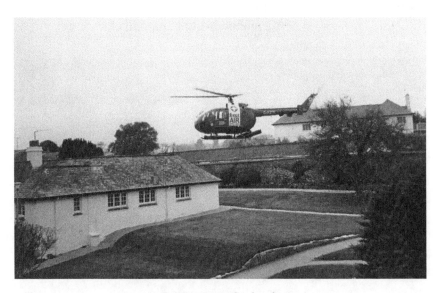

Figure 19 – Tango India landing at our
Truro City Hospital 'helipad'.

I went on to work in other parts of the helicopter industry as a pilot, consultant, instructor and manager in the North Sea, Ireland, Italy, The Netherlands, Brazil, Croatia, Spain, Canada, Cameroon, Russia and Malaysia. In 1990 I was tasked with re-establishing the functionality of the Strathclyde Police Air Support Unit following their fatal accident in January of that year.

I also worked as a Search and Rescue pilot in Ireland and was Chief Pilot of the London Air Ambulance for two years.

For most of the last ten years, I have been teaching at the AgustaWestland (now Leonardo Helicopters) Training Academy in Italy spending two weeks at work and then two weeks back home in Cornwall. Conceiving, designing and setting up this air ambulance unit was a truly life-changing experience during which I saw some of the best and perhaps some the worst of human nature. Anyone working at the sharp end of the emergency services would experience the same. Life in the emergency services is anything but dull. My abiding memory is of the professionalism and skill of my crew.

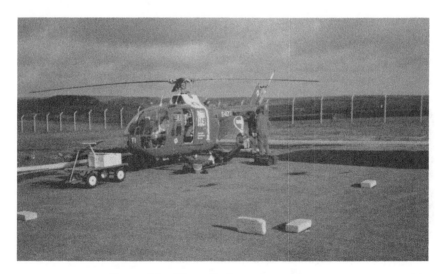

Figure 20 – Tango India is cleaned between
missions and prepared for the next callout.

My thanks to my wife, Lesley, for her never-ending belief in me and my crazy ideas. To Peter, my engineer for his commitment to our project, to Len Holden for handing me the opportunity that day in 1986, to Nigel Selwood who brought modern day thinking to pre-hospital care, and to all the friends and supporters who helped us through difficult times. This booklet tells an upbeat story, but it should not be forgotten that there were many tears shed during the days when things did not go according to plan. Thankfully the Cornwall Air Ambulance was just something that was destined to be. Now that I am semi-retired I have embarked on a new career as an author. My first four books were crime-thrillers, but other genres will also feature in the future. In the meantime, I continue to work as an instructor, advisor and consultant within the helicopter industry. Reading this account of the genesis of the Cornwall Air Ambulance is designed to encourage you to try my other books, I hope you will – they are all available on Amazon and other booksellers.

Information is also available at www.geoffnewman.co.uk

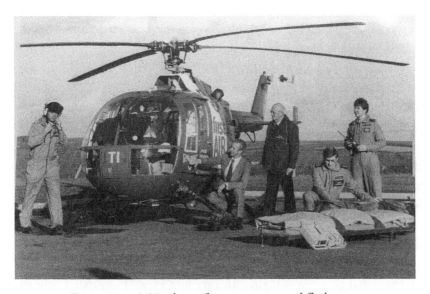

Figure 21 – A PR photo of management and flight crew.

41

INTERPRETING MY PILOT'S LOG

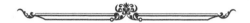

A professional pilot's log must be completed after each flight and must contain the data indicated at the top of each column. Most of the information is self-explanatory, but additional explanations are needed to ensure that entries are not misinterpreted.

Journey or Nature of Flight

In this column, I have detailed the point of departure, the point of arrival and any intermediate stops. Only rarely do I provide an exact landing point. It must be remembered that in 1987 the Truro A & E department was in the centre of the city with a tiny lawn area outside that could only be used for cases thought to be 'life-threatening'. It wasn't an easy landing site to get into particularly if the wind was southerly.

If we delivered a patient to Truro City A & E then we would normally land at CSSD, our regular parking and operating compound, we would be met by an ambulance and the patient transferred down to A & E. CSSD was the centralised sterilisation depot located at the top of the Treliske site with direct access to open country.

Our regional centre was Plymouth Freedom Fields Hospital. There was no helipad at the hospital so we would use the Freedom Fields Park next door. The local Fire Service unit would usually send a fire engine to stand by. Sometimes the patients transferred from Truro to Plymouth would be taken to the Airport for Derriford Hospital.

Mission

In this column, I have written either the task as passed to us on departure, the actual task as delivered or the best guess diagnosis available at the time. We often discovered more information later, but it was my habit to leave an entry as is. No entry should be taken as definitive. Only the clinicians that receive our patients can say for sure what the ultimate diagnosis was.

Flight Times

These are shown in hours and minutes. I do not use the decimal system in this log book.

© Geoff Newman

Year 1987 Month/Date	Aircraft Type	Registration	Commander	Holder's Operating Capacity	From (Dep)	To (Arr)	Times	Day Flying Pilot-in-Command (P1)	Co-Pilot (P2)	Dual	Night Flying Pilot-in-Command (P1)	Co-Pilot (P2)	Dual	Instrument Flying	Instructor	MISSION
							Totals carried forward	4033.55	1092.50	289.40	319.55	140.25	32.25	494.30	966.40	
Mar-20	MBB 105 DB	G-AZTI	SELF	P1			Bourn	0.10								Test Flight - vibro
Mar-21	MBB 105 DB	G-AZTI	SELF	P1			Bourn - St Mawgan	2.05								Delivery of first HEMS Helicopter Plus paramedic Paul Westaway and radio engineer Nigel Penton Tilbury
Mar-22	MBB 105 DB	G-AZTI	SELF	P1			St. Mawgan local	0.30								Media flight with TSW and Radio 4 Plus Paul Westaway and Bob Alderson
Mar-23	MBB 105 DB	G-AZTI	SELF	P1			St Mawgan - Truro	0.20								Opening ceremony. Plus Paul Westaway and Bob Alderson
Mar-23	MBB 105 DB	G-AZTI	SELF	P1			Truro local	0.05								Opening ceremony. Plus Paul Westaway and Bob Alderson
Mar-23	MBB 105 DB	G-AZTI	SELF	P1			Truro local	0.05								Reposition to our compound
Mar-24	MBB 105 DB	G-AZTI	SELF	P1			Truro local	0.05								Demo flight with paramedic Nigel Harris, Dr Nigel Selwood A&E Consultant and Ian Stewart
Mar-25	MBB 105 DB	G-AZTI	SELF	P1			Truro - Bodmin - St Mawgan - Bodmin - Truro	2.10								Crew Training
Mar-26	MBB 105 DB	G-AZTI	SELF	P1			Truro - Culdrose - Truro	3.00								Crew Training - visit to Dr Rick Jolly at Culdrose medical centre
Mar-30	MBB 105 DB	G-AZTI	SELF	P1			Truro local	0.15								Crew Training
Mar-30	MBB 105 DB	G-AZTI	SELF	P1			Truro - Carradon Hill - Davidstowe Moor - Carradon Hill	1.35								Crew Training

Year 1987 Month/Date	AIRCRAFT Type	Registration	Commander	Holder's Operating Capacity	Journey or Nature of Flight From (Dep) — To (Arr) (Times)	Day Flying Pilot-in-Command	Day Flying Co-Pilot (P2)	Dual	Night Flying Pilot-in-Command	Night Flying Co-Pilot (P2)	Dual	Instrument Flying	Instructor	MISSION
					Totals carried forward	4052.05	1092.50	289.40	319.55	140.25	32.25	494.30	966.40	
Apr-01	MBB 105 DB	G-AZTI	SELF	P1	Truro - Davistowe Moor Airfield - Porthcurnow - Truro	1.15								Mission 1 - Broken leg, local crew dealt with it. Mission 2 - Female student with back injury. Delivered to Treleiske
Apr-02	MBB 105 DB	G-AZTI	SELF	P1	Truro - Carnmenellis - Truro	0.10								Farmer with broken leg
Apr-03	MBB 105 DB	G-AZTI	SELF	P1	Truro - Bodmin - Truro	0.25								Patient-resuscitated by ground crew, taken to Treliske
Apr-03	MBB 105 DB	G-AZTI	SELF	P1	Truro - St Ives - Plymouth - Truro	1.10								Fisherman with hand injury
Apr-03	MBB 105 DB	G-AZTI	SELF	P1	Truro - Truro	0.10								False alarm
Apr-03	MBB 105 DB	G-AZTI	SELF	P1	Truro - Lostwithiel - Plymouth - Truro	0.45								RTC - 2 to Freedom Fields
Apr-04	MBB 105 DB	G-AZTI	SELF	P1	Truro - Mylor Bridge - Truro	0.10								Young boy in RTC, not serous, dealt with by road crew.
Apr-04	MBB 105 DB	G-AZTI	SELF	P1	Truro Wadebridge - Truro	0.20								2 horse-riders, one broken collar bone and one broken ribs
Apr-05	MBB 105 DB	G-AZTI	SELF	P1	Truro - St Austell - Truro	0.20								Footballer with broken leg
Apr-06	MBB 105 DB	G-AZTI	SELF	P1	Truro local	0.25								Air to Air photos with Richard Cook and Andrew Linklater
Apr-06	MBB 105 DB	G-AZTI	SELF	P1	Truro - St Austell - Truro	0.35								Suspected fractured femur
Apr-10	MBB 105 DB	G-AZTI	SELF	P1	Truro - Bude - Plymouth	0.35								Patient taken to Plymouth for urgent surgery
Apr-10	MBB 105 DB	G-AZTI	SELF	P1	Plymouth - St Columb - Truro	0.25								RTC - 2 to Treliske
Apr-11	MBB 105 DB	G-AZTI	SELF	P1	Truro Perranporth - Truro	0.10								Crashed hang glider
Apr-11	MBB 105 DB	G-AZTI	SELF	P1	Truro - Launceston - Plymouth	0.30								Motorcyclist - spinal injury
Apr-11	MBB 105 DB	G-AZTI	SELF	P1	Plymouth - Launceston - Plymouth	0.30								Appendicitis
Apr-11	MBB 105 DB	G-AZTI	SELF	P1	Plymouth - St Austell - Truro	0.20								Unconscious policeman after assault
Apr-12	MBB 105 DB	G-AZTI	SELF	P1	Truro - Mevagissey - Truro	0.15								Overdose
Apr-15	MBB 105 DB	G-AZTI	SELF	P1	Truro - St Mawes - Truro	0.15								Broken ankle

Year 1987 Month/Date	AIRCRAFT Type	Registration	Commander	Holder's Operating Capacity	Journey or Nature of Flight From (Dep)	To (Arr)	Day Flying Pilot-in-Command (P1)	Co-Pilot (P2)	Dual	Night Flying Pilot-in-Command (P1)	Co-Pilot (P2)	Dual	Instrument Flying	Instructor	MISSION
						Totals carried forward	4060.40	1092.50	289.40	319.55	140.25	32.25	494.30	966.40	
Apr-15	MBB 105 DB	G-AZTI	SELF	P1	Truro - Newquay - Truro		0.15								Broken collar bone and dislocated shoulder
Apr-15	MBB 105 DB	G-AZTI	SELF	P1	Truro - St Wenn - Truro		0.20								Spinal injuries
Apr-16	MBB 105 DB	G-AZTI	SELF	P1	Truro - Newquay - City Hospital A & E - CSSD		0.25								Man trapped by the leg under tractor. This was the first time we used the emergency landing site outside the A&E in Truro city hospital.
Apr-16	MBB 105 DB	G-AZTI	SELF	P1	Truro - Cothele Quay - Plymouth - Truro		1.00								Head injury - serious
Apr-17	MBB 105 DB	G-AZTI	SELF	P1	Truro - St Mary's - Penzance - Truro		1.00								Coronary
Apr-17	MBB 105 DB	G-AZTI	SELF	P1	Truro - Hightertown (Camelford) - Truro		0.30								Ladder fall - leg injury
Apr-17	MBB 105 DB	G-AZTI	SELF	P1	Truro - St Ives - Truro		0.20								Broken ankle on coastal path.
Apr-17	MBB 105 DB	G-AZTI	SELF	P1	Truro - Plymouth Freedom Fields - Truro		0.45								Inter-hospital transfer for neurosurgery
Apr-18	MBB 105 DB	G-AZTI	SELF	P1	Truro - Plymouth Airport - RNAS Culdrose		1.05								Kidney failure to Derriford
Apr-18	MBB 105 DB	G-AZTI	SELF	P1	RNAS Culdrose - City LZ Truro A & E		0.25								RTC - 5 year old boy
Apr-18	MBB 105 DB	G-AZTI	SELF	P1	City LZ - Plymouth Freedom Fields - Airport - Truro		0.35								5 year old boy to neurosurgery.
Apr-19	MBB 105 DB	G-AZTI	SELF	P1	Truro - Liskeard - Plymouth Airport - Truro		0.55								Elderly lady with emphasema
Apr-19	MBB 105 DB	G-AZTI	SELF	P1	Truro - Wadebridge - Truro		0.20								RTC - motorcyclist - no injury
Apr-20	MBB 105 DB	G-AZTI	SELF	P1	Truro - Treen (Lands End) - Truro		0.30								Coast path walker with broken ankle
Apr-23	MBB 105 DB	G-AZTI	SELF	P1	Truro - Liskeard - Culdrose - Truro		0.40								To Castle Air for nitrogen top-up then to patient with broken arm and cardiac problems
Apr-24	MBB 105 DB	G-AZTI	SELF	P1	Truro - Plymouth Freedom Fields - Airport - Davidstowe		0.45								Standby
Apr-24	MBB 105 DB	G-AZTI	SELF	P1	Davidstowe - Launcesto - Liskeard		0.15								Standby
Apr-24	MBB 105 DB	G-AZTI	SELF	P1	Liskeard - Padstow - Truro		0.20								?
Apr-25	MBB 105 DB	G-AZTI	SELF	P1	Truro - Mawnan Smith - Truro		0.15								?

Year 1987 Month/Date	AIRCRAFT Type	Registration	Commander	Holder's Operating Capacity	Journey or Nature of Flight From (Dep)	To (Arr)	(Times)	Day Flying Pilot-in-Command (P1)	Co-Pilot (P2)	Dual	Night Flying Pilot-in-Command (P1)	Co-Pilot (P2)	Dual	Instrument Flying	Instructor	MISSION
						Totals carried forward		4071.20	1092.50	289.40	319.55	140.25	32.25	494.3	966.4	
Apr-26	MBB 105 DB	G-AZTI	SELF	P1		Truro - Polzeath		0.25								Lacerated leg
Apr-26	MBB 105 DB	G-AZTI	SELF	P1		Polzeath - Goss Moor - City LZ		0.10								RTC 1 x Punctured lung, 1 x head and shoulder injuries
Apr-26	MBB 105 DB	G-AZTI	SELF	P1		City LZ - Newquay - Truro		0.10								Epileptic collapse
Apr-26	MBB 105 DB	G-AZTI	SELF	P1		Truro - Launceston - Plymouth Freedom Fields		0.35								Fractured elbow
Apr-26	MBB 105 DB	G-AZTI	SELF	P1		Freedom Fields - Port Isaac - Truro		0.25								Fractured ankle
Apr-27	MBB 105 DB	G-AZTI	SELF	P1		Truro - Ordstock Hospital (Hampshire) - Bournemouth Airport - Truro		2.35								Inter hospital transfer of paraplegic patient. C3 fracture after diving into sea that was too shallow.
Apr-27	MBB 105 DB	G-AZTI	SELF	P1		Truro - St Tuddy - Tehidy - Truro		0.35								Stroke patient
Apr-27	MBB 105 DB	G-AZTI	SELF	P1		Truro - Falmouth - Truro		0.10								Baby with fat burns
Apr-30	MBB 105 DB	G-AZTI	SELF	P1		Truro - Lostwithiel - Truro		0.35								Neck injury
Apr-30	MBB 105 DB	G-AZTI	SELF	P1		Truro - Bodmin		0.05								No injury RTC
Apr-30	MBB 105 DB	G-AZTI	SELF	P1		Bodmin - Blisland - Truro		0.20								Urgent medical care required
May-01	MBB 105 DB	G-AZTI	SELF	P1		Truro - Plymouth Airport		0.25								Man with flash burns received whilst working in a car servicing pit.
May-01	MBB 105 DB	G-AZTI	SELF	P1		Plymouth Airport to Delabole		0.15								Heart attack
May-01	MBB 105 DB	G-AZTI	SELF	P1		Delabole - Launceston - Plymouth Freedom Fields		0.20								Spinal injuries
May-01	MBB 105 DB	G-AZTI	SELF	P1		Plymouth Freedom Fields - Castle Air - Delabole - Freedom Fields - Truro		1.00								Lung cancer
May-02	MBB 105 DB	G-AZTI	SELF	P1		Truro - Polzeath - Truro		0.25								Heart attack
May-02	MBB 105 DB	G-AZTI	SELF	P1		Truro - St Mawgan - Truro		0.10								Broken wrist and back injuries
May-02	MBB 105 DB	G-AZTI	SELF	P1		Truro - Porthleven - Truro		0.10								Leg fracture
May-02	MBB 105 DB	G-AZTI	SELF	P1		Truro - Plymouth Airport - Truro		0.50								Inter hospital transfer - Kidney failure

Year 1987 Month/Date	AIRCRAFT Type	Registration	Commander	Holder's Operating Capacity	Journey or Nature of Flight From (Dep)	To (Arr)	Day Flying Pilot-in-Command (P1)	Co-Pilot (P2)	Dual	Night Flying Pilot-in-Command (P1)	Co-Pilot (P2)	Dual	Instrument Flying	Instructor	MISSION
					Totals carried forward		4080.50	1092.50	289.40	319.55	140.25	32.25	494.30	966.40	
May-03	MBB 105 DB	G-AZTI	SELF	P1	Truro - Bude - Plymouth		0.40								Urgent medical transfer
May-03	MBB 105 DB	G-AZTI	SELF	P1	Plymouth - Truro		0.20								Premature birth
May-03	MBB 105 DB	G-AZTI	SELF	P1	Truro - Plymouth FF - Truro		0.40								Fractured skull
May-03	MBB 105 DB	G-AZTI	SELF	P1	Truro - Penzance - Truro		0.30								Fractured leg
May-04	MBB 105 DB	G-AZTI	SELF	P1	Truro - Helstone - Truro		0.40								Asthma attack
May-04	MBB 105 DB	G-AZTI	SELF	P1	Truro - Mullion Golf Club - Truro		0.15								Head injury after being struck by golf ball
May-07	MBB 105 DB	G-AZTI	SELF	P1	Truro - Delabole - Truro		0.30								Brain bleed
May-07	MBB 105 DB	G-AZTI	SELF	P1	Truro - Watergate Bay - Truro		0.15								Head injuries
May-07	MBB 105 DB	G-AZTI	SELF	P1	Truro - Plymounth - Truro		0.45								Burns (covered in hot pitch)
May-07	MBB 105 DB	G-AZTI	SELF	P1	Truro - Polruan - St Austell - Plymouth		0.35								Traumatic amputation of hand whilst changing saw blade
May-07	MBB 105 DB	G-AZTI	SELF	P1	Plymouth - Polruan - Exeter		0.45								Renal failure
May-07	MBB 105 DB	G-AZTI	SELF	P1	Exeter - Plymouth FF - Truro		0.40								Brain bleed
May-08	MBB 105 DB	G-AZTI	SELF	P1	Truro - Davidstowe - Plymouth - Castle Air - Truro		0.50								Pneumonia
May-08	MBB 105 DB	G-AZTI	SELF	P1	Truro - St Marys - Truro		1.00								Fractured femur
May-09	MBB 105 DB	G-AZTI	SELF	P1	Truro - Manaccan - Truro		0.10								Chest injuries
May-10	MBB 105 DB	G-AZTI	SELF	P1	Truro - Newquay - Truro		0.15								Baby with heart problems
May-14	MBB 105 DB	G-AZTI	SELF	P1	Truro - RNAS Culdrose		0.25								Baby (drowning)
May-15	MBB 105 DB	G-AZTI	SELF	P1	Truro - Castle Air - Davidstowe		0.30								Top-up nitrogen in the float bottles
May-15	MBB 105 DB	G-AZTI	SELF	P1	Davidstowe - Gorran - Truro		0.25								Fractured ankle

Year 1987 Month/Date	AIRCRAFT Type	Registration	Commander	Holder's Operating Capacity	Journey or Nature of Flight From (Dep)	To (Arr)	Day Flying Pilot-In-Command	Co-Pilot (P2)	Dual	Night Flying Pilot-In-Command	Co-Pilot (P2)	Dual	Instrument Flying	Instructor	MISSION
					Totals carried forward		4092.50	1092.50	289.40	319.55	140.25	32.25	494.30	966.40	
May-16	MBB 105 DB	G-AZTI	SELF	P1	Truro - St Breward - Truro		0.20								Stroke
May-16	MBB 105 DB	G-AZTI	SELF	P1	Truro - Watergate Bay - Ladock - Truro		0.30								Cricketer with epilepsy and back injury
May-17	MBB 105 DB	G-AZTI	SELF	P1	Truro - Penzance - Plymouth - Truro		1.15								Head injury
May-18	MBB 105 DB	G-AZTI	SELF	P1	Truro - Madron - Truro		0.20								Man fell down mine shaft whilst retrieving stolen motorcycle parts injuring his spine and legs. Retrieved courtesy of the Fire Service and our paramedic.
May-21	MBB 105 DB	G-AZTI	SELF	P1	Truro - Penzance - St Mawgan - Truro		0.40								Delivery of heart bypass patient to fixed wing air ambulance
May-22	MBB 105 DB	G-AZTI	SELF	P1	Truro - Penzance - Plymouth Airport - Bodmin - Truro		1.10								Baby with scalding
May-23	MBB 105 DB	G-AZTI	SELF	P1	Truro - Mylor Harbour - Truro		0.10								Plane crash. Schneider trophy replica seaplane suffered tail flutter and crashed beside Mylor Creek. Fatal.
May-24	MBB 105 DB	G-AZTI	SELF	P1	Truro - Leryn - Bodmin		0.20								Patient deceased. Mission aborted.
May-24	MBB 105 DB	G-AZTI	SELF	P1	Bodmin - Golant - Plymouth FF - Bodmin Airfield		0.35								Head injuries
May-24	MBB 105 DB	G-AZTI	SELF	P1	Bodmin A/F - Newquay - Truro		0.15								Pelvic and internal injuries
May-25	MBB 105 DB	G-AZTI	SELF	P1	Truro - Hayle - Truro		0.20								Leg injuries
May-25	MBB 105 DB	G-AZTI	SELF	P1	Truro - Bodmin - Truro		0.30								Carcenoma
May-28	MBB 105 DB	G-AZTI	SELF	P1	Truro - Plymouth FF - Bodmin A/F		0.45								Hydrocephalus
May-28	MBB 105 DB	G-AZTI	SELF	P1	Bodmin A/F - Truro		0.15								Collapse in Portscatho - mission aborted - RTB
May-29	MBB 105 DB	G-AZTI	SELF	P1	Truro - Penzance - Plymouth Dive Centre - Truro		1.45								Diver with bends delivered to the dive centre located in the old Napoleonic Fort
May-30	MBB 105 DB	G-AZTI	SELF	P1	Truro - local		0.15								Chairman of the DHA - PR.
May-30	MBB 105 DB	G-AZTI	SELF	P1	Truro - St Austell		0.10								Positioning
May-30	MBB 105 DB	G-AZTI	SELF	P1	Truro - City LZ - Plymouth - Truro		1.00								Head injury. Urgent transfer to neurosurgery
May-31	MBB 105 DB	G-AZTI	SELF	P1	Truro Mullion - City LZ - CSSD		0.25								Spinal injury

Year 1987 Month/Date	AIRCRAFT		Commander	Holder's Operating Capacity	Journey or Nature of Flight		Day Flying			Night Flying			Instrument Flying	Instructor	MISSION
	Type	Registration			From (Dep)	To (Arr)	Pilot-in-Command	Co-Pilot (P2)	Dual	Pilot-in-Command	Co-Pilot (P2)	Dual			
					Totals carried forward		4102.00	1092.50	289.40	319.55	140.25	32.25	494.3	966.4	
May-31	MBB 105 DB	G-AZTI	SELF	P1	Truro - Fraddon - Truro		0.10								Compound fracture of Tib & Fib
May-31	MBB 105 DB	G-AZTI	SELF	P1	Truro - St Austell - truro		0.15								Position to traction engine rally - on standby
Jun-01	MBB 105 DB	G-AZTI	SELF	P1	Truro - Liskeard - Bodmin		0.20								Recharge nitrogen
Jun-01	MBB 105 DB	G-AZTI	SELF	P1	Bodmin - Polzeath - Truro		0.15								Broken ankle
Jun-01	MBB 105 DB	G-AZTI	SELF	P1	Truro - Newquay - Truro		0.10								Heart attack
Jun-04	MBB 105 DB	G-AZTI	SELF	P1	Truro - Wadebridge - St Buryan - Redruth - Truro		0.50								Medical emergency
Jun-05	MBB 105 DB	G-AZTI	SELF	P1	Truro - Wadebridge - St Merryn - Truro		0.25								To Royal Show the RTC - 2 patients with leg and head injuries
Jun-05	MBB 105 DB	G-AZTI	SELF	P1	Truro - Wadebridge Royal Showground		0.15								To Royal Show on standby
Jun-05	MBB 105 DB	G-AZTI	SELF	P1	Showground - Dobwalls - Truro		0.50								To RTC at Dobwalls. Return flight aborted due weather - fog
Jun-06	MBB 105 DB	G-AZTI	SELF	P1	Truro - Wadebridge Royal Showground		0.10								To Royal Show on standby
Jun-06	MBB 105 DB	G-AZTI	SELF	P1	Showground - Truro		0.20								RTB
Jun-07	MBB 105 DB	G-AZTI	SELF	P1	Truro - Callington - Plymouth FF - Truro		0.45								Leg injury
Jun-07	MBB 105 DB	G-AZTI	SELF	P1	Truro - Perranporth - Truro		0.10								Dr Simcox - training flight
Jun-07	MBB 105 DB	G-AZTI	SELF	P1	Truro - Lockengate - Truro		0.20								Young boy injured competing in motorcycle scramble.
Jun-08	MBB 105 DB	G-AZTI	SELF	P1	Truro - Bude - Plymouth - Truro		0.55								Inner ear infection
Jun-11	MBB 105 DB	G-AZTI	SELF	P1	Truro - Gweek - Truro		0.15								Motorcyclist with query fractured knee cap
Jun-11	MBB 105 DB	G-AZTI	SELF	P1	Truro - Helston - Truro		0.15								young girl injured at Aero Park + adult (teacher)
Jun-11	MBB 105 DB	G-AZTI	SELF	P1	Truro - The Lizard - Truro		0.25								Elderly patient with pneumonia
Jun-11	MBB 105 DB	G-AZTI	SELF	P1	Truro - Week St Mary - Plymouth FF - Liskeard - Truro		0.55								Elderly patient with urgent medical condition

Year 1987 Month/Date	AIRCRAFT		Commander	Holder's Operating Capacity	Journey or Nature of Flight		Day Flying			Night Flying			Instrument Flying	Instructor	MISSION
	Type	Registration			From (Dep)	To (Arr)	Pilot-in-Command	Co-Pilot (P2)	Dual	Pilot-in-Command	Co-Pilot (P2)	Dual			
					Totals carried forward		4110.00	1092.50	289.40	319.55	140.25	32.25	494.30	966.40	
Jun-13	MBB 105 DB	G-AZTI	SELF	P1	Truro - Rejerrah - Truro		0.10								RTC - Leg and head injuries
Jun-13	MBB 105 DB	G-AZTI	SELF	P1	Truro - Zelah - City LZ - CSSD		0.15								RTC - motorcyclist severe leg injuries
Jun-13	MBB 105 DB	G-AZTI	SELF	P1	Truro - Leedstown - Truro		0.10								RTC - 2 patients with minor injuries
Jun-14	MBB 105 DB	G-AZTI	SELF	P1	Truro - Plymouth Airport - Delabole		0.40								Badly burnt baby + mother to burns unit. (campsite gas burner flash fire
Jun-14	MBB 105 DB	C-AZTI	SELF	P1	Delabole - Truro		0.15								Brain injury
Jun-14	MBB 105 DB	G-AZTI	SELF	P1	Truro - Polkerris - Truro		0.20								Stroke
Jun-14	MBB 105 DB	G-AZTI	SELF	P1	Truro - Gurnards Head - Truro		0.25								Broken ankle
Jun-14	MBB 105 DB	G-AZTI	SELF	P1	Truro - Par - Truro		0.15								Collapse
Jun-18	MBB 105 DB	G-AZTI	SELF	P1	Truro - Plymouth FF - Truro		0.50								Aortic aneurism and renal failure
Jun-19	MBB 105 DB	G-AZTI	SELF	P1	Truro - St Breward - Truro		0.30								Broken ankle
Jun-19	MBB 105 DB	G-AZTI	SELF	P1	Truro - St Austell - Truro		0.15								Severe medical condition - abdominal
Jun-20	MBB 105 DB	G-AZTI	SELF	P1	Truro - Plymouth FF - Bodmin		0.40								Chuild with brain injury
Jun-20	MBB 105 DB	G-AZTI	SELF	P1	Bodmin - Keley Brae - Plymouth FF - Airport - Bodmin		0.40								Male with heart dysrhymia
Jun-20	MBB 105 DB	G-AZTI	SELF	P1	Bodmin - East Restormel - City LZ - CSSD		0.20								2 x motorcyclists with multiple injuries.
Jun-20	MBB 105 DB	G-AZTI	SELF	P1	Truro local		0.25								Mission aborted
Jun-21	MBB 105 DB	G-AZTI	SELF	P1	Truro St Mawgan - Truro		0.10								Injured footballer
Jun-21	MBB 105 DB	G-AZTI	SELF	P1	Truro - Mylor - Truro		0.10								Patient with head, arm and leg injuries
Jun-21	MBB 105 DB	G-AZTI	SELF	P1	Truro - Plymouth FF		0.15								Stab victim with paralysis
Jun-21	MBB 105 DB	G-AZTI	SELF	P1	Plymouth - St Merryn - City LZ - CSSD		0.35								Parachutist with smashed legs

Year 1987 Month/Date	AIRCRAFT Type	Registration	Commander	Holder's Operating Capacity	From (Dep)	(Times)	To (Arr)	Pilot-in-Command	Co-Pilot (P2)	Dual	Pilot-in-Command	Co-Pilot (P2)	Dual	Instrument Flying	Instructor	MISSION
						Totals carried forward			1092.50	289.40	319.55	140.25	32.25	494.30	966.40	
Jun-22	MBB 105 DB	G-AZTI	SELF	P1	Truro - Fowey - Truro			0.25								Korean seaman hit by hatch cover
Jun-25	MBB 105 DB	G-AZTI	SELF	P1	Truro - Praze - Truro			0.20								RTC - assisted ground crews
Jun-26	MBB 105 DB	G-AZTI	SELF	P1	Truro - Bude - Barnstable - Truro			1.35								Lacerated legs
Jun-27	MBB 105 DB	G-AZTI	SELF	P1	Truro local			0.30								To - Post Grad Centre, To ST Austell and return
Jun-29	MBB 105 DB	G-AZTI	SELF	P1	Truro - Liskeard - Bodmin			0.20								To Castle Air
Jun-29	MBB 105 DB	G-AZTI	SELF	P1	Bodmin - St Columb Road - Truro			0.15								Medical admission
Jul-02	MBB 105 DB	G-AZTI	SELF	P1	Truro - St Breward - Truro			0.30								Broken arm
Jul-02	MBB 105 DB	G-AZTI	SELF	P1	Truro Sennen - City LZ - CSSD			0.35								Man with traumatic amputation of toes after argument with lawn mower
Jul-02	MBB 105 DB	G-AZTI	SELF	P1	Truro - Ruan Minor - City LZ - CSSD			0.20								7 year old boy - RTC - head and leg injuries
Jul-03	MBB 105 DB	G-AZTI	SELF	P1	Truro - St Eval - Truro			0.20								Head injury
Jul-03	MBB 105 DB	G-AZTI	SELF	P1	Truro - Port Isaac - Truro			0.30								Riding accident - head injury
Jul-03	MBB 105 DB	G-AZTI	SELF	P1	Truro - Delabole - Truro			0.30								Heart attack
Jul-04	MBB 105 DB	G-AZTI	SELF	P1	Truro local			0.15								Power assurance check
Jul-04	MBB 105 DB	G-AZTI	SELF	P1	Truro local			0.10								Mission aborted
Jul-04	MBB 105 DB	G-AZTI	SELF	P1	Truro - Looe - Plymouth FF - Airport			0.40								Head injury
Jul-04	MBB 105 DB	G-AZTI	SELF	P1	Plymouth Airport - Bude - Plymouth FF			0.30								Leg injury
Jul-04	MBB 105 DB	G-AZTI	SELF	P1	FF - Truro			0.15								Hospital transfer
Jul-05	MBB 105 DB	G-AZTI	SELF	P1	Truro Week St Mary - Hayle			0.45								Collapse
Jul-05	MBB 105 DB	G-AZTI	SELF	P1	Hayle - Truro			0.10								Collapse

Year 1987 Month/Date	AIRCRAFT		Commander	Holder's Operating Capacity	Journey or Nature of Flight		Day Flying			Night Flying			Instrument Flying	Instructor	MISSION
	Type	Registration			From (Dep)	To (Arr) (Times)	Pilot-in-Command	Co-Pilot (P2)	Dual	Pilot-in-Command	Co-Pilot (P2)	Dual			
					Totals carried forward		4124.10	1092.50	289.40	319.55	140.25	32.25	494.30	966.40	
Jul-05	MBB 105 DB	G-AZTI	SELF	P1	Truro - Ianteglos - Truro		0.30								Acute abdominal pains
Jul-05	MBB 105 DB	G-AZTI	SELF	P1	Truro - Tredrizzick - Truro		0.20								Urgent medical condition
Jul-05	MBB 105 DB	G-AZTI	SELF	P1	Truro - Delabole - Truro		0.30								Unconscious
Jul-06	MBB 105 DB	G-AZTI	SELF	P1	Truro - Bodmin - City LZ - CSSD		0.25								Laceraions to the neck
Jul-06	MBB 105 DB	G-AZTI	SELF	P1	Truro - St Dennis - Truro		0.10								RTC - Head injuries
Jul-09	MBB 105 DB	G-AZTI	SELF	P1	Truro - Cardinham - Bodmin		0.20								RTC - Motorcyclist with leg injuries
Jul-09	MBB 105 DB	G-AZTI	SELF	P1	Bodmin - Truro		0.15								RTC - Query attempted suicide
Jul-09	MBB 105 DB	G-AZTI	SELF	P1	Truro - The Lizard - Truro		0.20								Broken ankle
Jul-10	MBB 105 DB	G-ZZTI	SELF	P1	Truro - Penzance - Plymouth FF - Airport		0.45								Brain bleed
Jul-10	MBB 105 DB	G-FZTI	SELF	P1	Airport - Penzance - Truro		0.40								Brain bleed
Jul-10	MBB 105 DB	G-AZTI	SELF	P1	Truro - Portscatho - Truro		0.10								Acute airway obstuction
Jul-10	MBB 105 DB	G-AZTI	SELF	P1	Truro - St Austell - Truro		0.20								RTC - no injury
Jul-10	MBB 105 DB	G-AZTI	SELF	P1	Truro - Rock - Plymouth FF - Truro		0.25			0.25					RTC
Jul-11	MBB 105 DB	G-AZTI	SELF	P1	Truro - Par - Truro		0.20								RTC - head arm and leg injuries
Jul-12	MBB 105 DB	G-AZTI	SELF	P1	Truro - Lands End - Truro		0.35								Broken ankle
Jul-12	MBB 105 DB	G-AZTI	SELF	P1	Truro - Fowey - Truro		0.15								Leg wound
Jul-12	MBB 105 DB	G-AZTI	SELF	P1	Truro - Hayle - Truro		0.10								Concussion
Jul-12	MBB 105 DB	G-AZTI	SELF	P1	Truro - Caesand - Plymouth - Truro		1.00								Hypothermia
Jul-13	MBB 105 DB	G-AZTI	SELF	P1	Truro - Bodmin - Bodmin A/F - Truro		0.30								PR Visit to St Mary's School

Year 1987 Month/Date	AIRCRAFT Type	Registration	Commander	Holder's Operating Capacity	Journey or Nature of Flight From (Dep)	To (Arr)	(Times)	Day Flying Pilot-in-Command	Co-Pilot (P2)	Dual	Night Flying Pilot-in-Command	Co-Pilot (P2)	Dual	Instrument Flying	Instructor	MISSION
					Totals carried forward			4132.10	1092.50	289.40	320.20	140.25	32.25	494.30	966.40	
Jul-16	MBB 105 DB	G-AZTI	SELF	P1	Truro local test flight			0.05								n/a
Jul-16	MBB 105 DB	G-AZTI	SELF	P1	Truro - Percuil - Truro			0.15								Broken ankle
Jul-16	MBB 105 DB	G-AZTI	SELF	P1	Truro - Kestle Mill - Truro			0.10								Multiple injuries
Jul-16	MBB 105 DB	G-AZTI	SELF	P1	Truro - Mevagissy - Truro			0.15								Renal cholic
Jul-17	MBB 105 DB	G-AZTI	SELF	P1	Truro - Week St Mary - Plymouth FF - Castle Air			0.30								Pregnant woman with abdominal pains
Jul-17	MBB 105 DB	G-AZTI	SELF	P1	Castle Air - Camelford - Truro			0.25								Infant with medical condition + mum
Jul-17	MBB 105 DB	G-AZTI	SELF	P1	Truro - Davidstowe - Bodmin A/F			0.30								Collapse
Jul-17	MBB 105 DB	G-AZTI	SELF	P1	Bodmin A/F - Polzeath - Truro			0.35								RTC
Jul-18	MBB 105 DB	G-AZTI	SELF	P1	Truro - Launceston - Plymouth Airport			0.30								traumatic amputation of ear by horse
Jul-18	MBB 105 DB	G-AZTI	SELF	P1	Plymouth Airport - Millbrook - St Austell			0.15								Terminal cancer
Jul-18	MBB 105 DB	G-AZTI	SELF	P1	St Austell - The Lizard - Truro			0.30								Broken ankle
Jul-18	MBB 105 DB	G-AZTI	SELF	P1	Truro - Newlyn - Truro			0.25								Dislocated fracture of the knee
Jul-20	MBB 105 DB	G-AZTI	SELF	P1	Truro - Falmouth - Truro			0.20								Heart attack
Jul-20	MBB 105 DB	G-AZTI	SELF	P1	Truro - Launceston - Plymouth FF - Truro			1.05								Medical condition
Jul-23	MBB 105 DB	G-AZTI	SELF	P1	Truro - Newquay - Truro			0.15								Heart attack
Jul-23	MBB 105 DB	G-AZTI	SELF	P1	Truro - Launceston - Plymouth FF - Airport - Bodmin			0.55								Broken leg (femur)
Jul-23	MBB 105 DB	G-AZTI	SELF	P1	Bodmin - Boscastle - Bodmin			0.20								Collapse - no transport required
Jul-23	MBB 105 DB	G-AZTI	SELF	P1	Bodmin - Davidstowe Moor - Plymouth FF			0.25								Head injury
Jul-23	MBB 105 DB	G-AZTI	SELF	P1	FF - Gorran Haven - Truro			0.25								Stroke

Year 1987 Month/Date	AIRCRAFT Type	Registration	Commander	Holder's Operating Capacity	Journey or Nature of Flight From (Dep)	To (Arr)	Day Flying Pilot-in-Command	Co-Pilot (P2)	Dual	Night Flying Pilot-in-Command	Co-Pilot (P2)	Dual	Instrument Flying	Instructor	MISSION
					Totals carried forward		4132.10	1092.50	289.40	320.20	140.25	32.25	494.30	966.40	
Jul-24	MBB 105 DB	G-AZTI	SELF	P1	Truro - Tintagel - Plymouth FF - Liskeard		0.50								Heart attack
Jul-24	MBB 105 DB	G-AZTI	SELF	P1	Liskeard - Hayle - Plymouth FF - Airport - Bodmin		1.10								To neurosurgeons query brain tumour
Jul-24	MBB 105 DB	G-AZTI	SELF	P1	Bodmin - Newquay - Truro		0.15								Horse rider accident
Jul-24	MBB 105 DB	G-AZTI	SELF	P1	Truro - Luxillian - Truro		0.15								Leg injury after contact with farm machinery
Jul-24	MBB 105 DB	G-AZTI	SELF	P1	Truro - Kilkhampton - Plymouth Airport - Truro		1.10								Severe abdominal pains
Jul-25	MBB 105 DB	G-AZTI	SELF	P1	Truro - Wendron - Truro		0.10								Publican at the New Inn fell down stairs - multiple injuries
Jul-25	MBB 105 DB	G-AZTI	SELF	P1	Truro - Tregony - Truro		0.10								Severe facial injuries
Jul-25	MBB 105 DB	G-AZTI	SELF	P1	Truro - St Kew Highway - Truro		0.30								Back injury
Jul-25	MBB 105 DB	G-AZTI	SELF	P1	Truro - Tintagel - Truro		0.30								Heart attack
Jul-26	MBB 105 DB	G-AZTI	SELF	P1	Truro - Delabole - Truro		0.25								Medical emergency
Jul-26	MBB 105 DB	G-AZTI	SELF	P1	Truro - Falmouth - Truro		0.10								Head injury
Jul-26	MBB 105 DB	G-AZTI	SELF	P1	Truro - Kuggar - City LZ - CSSD		0.20								Head and internal injuries
Jul-26	MBB 105 DB	G-AZTI	SELF	P1	Truro - Porthoustock - Truro		0.15								Heart attack
Jul-29	MBB 105 DB	G-AZTI	SELF	P1	Truro - Launceston - Plymouth FF - Airport - Bodmin A/F		0.40								Medical emergency
Jul-29	MBB 105 DB	G-AZTI	SELF	P1	Bodmin A/F - London Apprentice - Truro		0.15								RTC - no injury
Jul-30	MBB 105 DB	G-AZTI	SELF	P1	Truro - Launceston - Plymouth FF - Truro		0.55								Arm injuries
Jul-30	MBB 105 DB	G-AZTI	SELF	P1	Truro - St Mawgan - Truro		0.10								Heart attack
Jul-30	MBB 105 DB	G-AZTI	SELF	P1	Truro - Mevagissey - Truro		0.10								Non infectious meningitus
Jul-31	MBB 105 DB	G-AZTI	SELF	P1	Truro - Helston - Truro		0.10								Heart attack

Year 1987 Month/Date	AIRCRAFT Type	Registration	Commander	Holder's Operating Capacity	Journey or Nature of Flight From (Dep)	To (Arr) (Times)	Day Flying Pilot-in-Command	Co-Pilot (P2)	Dual	Night Flying Pilot-in-Command	Co-Pilot (P2)	Dual	Instrument Flying	Instructor	MISSION
					Totals carried forward		4149.50	1092.50	289.40	320.20	140.25	32.25	494.30	966.40	
Jul-31	MBB 105 DB	G-AZTI	SELF	P1	Truro Local		0.05								Weather Recce
Aug-01	MBB 105 DB	G-AZTI	SELF	P1	Truro - Davidstowe - Plymouth Airport		0.40								Renal colic
Aug-01	MBB 105 DB	G-AZTI	SELF	P1	Plymouth Apt - Tintagel - Plymouth Apt		0.35								Sub Arachnoid Haemorage
Aug-01	MBB 105 DB	G-AZTI	SELF	P1	Plymouth Apt - Tintagel - Plymouth FF - Airport		0.35								Fractured leg and head injuries
Aug-01	MBB 105 DB	G-AZTI	SELF	P1	Plymouth Apt - Polzeath - Truro		0.30								Dislocated shoulder
Aug-01	MBB 105 DB	G-AZTI	SELF	P1	Truro - Hayle - Truro		0.15								Head injuries and broken arm
Aug-01	MBB 105 DB	G-AZTI	SELF	P1	Truro - Rejearrah - Plymouth Apt - Truro		0.40								Burns
Aug-02	MBB 105 DB	G-AZTI	SELF	P1	Truro Local		0.20							Harris/Prissell	Filming
Aug-02	MBB 105 DB	G-AZTI	SELF	P1	Truro - Perranporth - Truro		0.10							Harris/Prissell	Drowning x2
Aug-05	MBB 105 DB	G-AZTI	SELF	P1	Truro - Plymouth FF - Launceston		0.3							Harris/Prissell	Brain Tumour
Aug-05	MBB 105 DB	G-AZTI	SELF	P1	Launceston - Newquay - Truro		0.20							Harris/Prissell	Myocardial infarction
Aug-06	MBB 105 DB	G-AZTI	SELF	P1	Truro - Bude - Plymouth FF - Apt		0.40							Harris/Prissell	Fractured Skull
Aug-06	MBB 105 DB	G-AZTI	SELF	P1	Plymouth Apt - St Mawgan village - Truro		0.25							Harris/Prissell	Fractured Femur
Aug-06	MBB 105 DB	G-AZTI	SELF	P1	Truro - Tintagel - Plymouth FF - Apt		0.40							Harris/Prissell	Stroke
Aug-06	MBB 105 DB	G-AZTI	SELF	P1	Plymouth Apt - Bude		0.15							Harris/Prissell	Fractured Skull
Aug-06	MBB 105 DB	G-AZTI	SELF	P1	Bude - Bodmin - Truro		0.25							Harris/Prissell	Head Injury
Aug-07	MBB 105 DB	G-AZTI	SELF	P1	Truro - Bodmin - Truro		.20							Harris/Prissell	RTA
Aug-07	MBB 105 DB	G-AZTI	SELF	P1	Truro - Veryan - Truro		0.10							Harris/Prissell	Broken Ankle on rocks
Aug-07	MBB 105 DB	G-AZTI	SELF	P1	Truro - St Mawgan - Bodmin - Truro		0.30							Harris/Prissell	Chest infection

Year 1987 Month/Date	AIRCRAFT Type	Registration	Commander	Holder's Operating Capacity	From (Dep)	To (Arr)	Day Flying Pilot-in-Command	Co-Pilot (P2)	Dual	Night Flying Pilot-in-Command	Co-Pilot (P2)	Dual	Instrument Flying	Instructor	MISSION	
					Totals carried forward		4157.55	1092.50	289.40	320.20	140.25	32.25	494.30	966.40		
Aug-07	MBB 105 DB	G-AZTI	SELF	P1	Truro - Wadebridge - Truro		0.30								Arterial Effusion	Harris/Prissell
Aug-07	MBB 105 DB	G-AZTI	SELF	P1	Truro - Bodmin - Plymouth FF - Apt - Truro		0.45								Multiple injuries	Harris/Prissell
Aug-08	MBB 105 DB	G-AZTI	SELF	P1	Truro - Mylor - Truro		0.10								CVA	Harris/Prissell
Aug-08	MBB 105 DB	G-AZTI	SELF	P1	Truro - Rock - Plymouth FF		0.30								Brain Tumour	Harris/Prissell
Aug-08	MBB 105 DB	G-AZTI	SELF	P1	Plymouth FF - Millbrook - Plymouth Apt		0.10								RTA - no injury	Harris/Prissell
Aug-08	MBB 105 DB	G-AZTI	SELF	P1	Plymouth Apt - Frogpool - Truro		0.40								Football head injury	Harris/Prissell
Aug-08	MBB 105 DB	G-AZTI	SELF	P1	Truro Local		0.30								PR, Porth Navas	Harris/Prissell
Aug-09	MBB 105 DB	G-AZTI	SELF	P1	Truro - Bude - Plymouth FF - Apt - Truro		0.45								Pulmonary embolysom	Westaway/Alderson
Aug-09	MBB 105 DB	G-AZTI	SELF	P1	Truro - Launceston - Barnstable - Truro		1.10								Lacerated knee	Westaway/Alderson
Aug-09	MBB 105 DB	G-AZTI	SELF	P1	Truro - Mullion - Truro		0.20								Septacaemia	Alderson/Slade
Aug-09	MBB 105 DB	G-AZTI	SELF	P1	Truro - Launceston - Plymouth FF - Truro		0.50								Fractured Leg	Alderson/Slade
Aug-09	MBB 105 DB	G-AZTI	SELF	P1	Truro - Perranporth - Truro		0.10								Facial Lacerations	Alderson/Slade
Aug-12	MBB 105 DB	G-AZTI	SELF	P1	Truro - Falmouth - Truro		0.10								Coronary (fatal)	Alderson/Slade
Aug-12	MBB 105 DB	G-AZTI	SELF	P1	Truro - Camelford - Truro		0.25								Coranary	Alderson/Slade
Aug-13	MBB 105 DB	G-AZTI	SELF	P1	Truro - Bude - Barnstable - Truro		1.20								Peritonitis	Alderson/Slade
Aug-13	MBB 105 DB	G-AZTI	SELF	P1	Truro - Wellcome - Barnstable - Truro		1.10								Dislocated Hip	Alderson/Slade
Aug-14	MBB 105 DB	G-AZTI	SELF	P1	Truro - Padstow - Truro		0.25								Dislocated knee	Bond Alderson/Westaway
Aug-14	MBB 105 DB	G-AZTI	SELF	P1	Truro - Bude - Plymouth FF - Apt - Truro		1.00								?	Alderson/Westaway
Sep-03	MBB 105 DB	G-AZTI	SELF	P1	Truro - Padstow - City - CSSD		0.25								Back Injury	Alderson/O'Byrne

Year 1987 Month/Date	Type	Registration	Commander	Holder's Operating Capacity	From (Dep)	To (Arr)	Times	Pilot-In-Command	Co-Pilot (P2)	Dual	Pilot-In-Command	Co-Pilot (P2)	Dual	Instrument Flying	Instructor	MISSION
					Totals carried forward			4169.20	1092.50	289.40	320.20	140.25	32.25	494.3	966.40	
Sep-04	MBB 105 DB	G-AZTI	SELF	P1	Truro - Bodmin - Truro			0.20								Miocardial Infarction Alderson/O'Byrne
Sep-04	MBB 105 DB	G-AZTI	SELF	P1	Truro - Sennen - Truro			0.35								Fractured & Dislocated Arm and Elbow Alderson/O'Byrne
Sep-04	MBB 105 DB	G-AZTI	SELF	P1	Truro - Bude - Plymouth FF			0.40								Fractured femur Alderson/O'Byrne
Sep-04	MBB 105 DB	G-AZTI	SELF	P1	Apt - Winnards Perch - City - CSSD			0.30								Lacerated leg and fractured femur Alderson/O'Byrne
Sep-05	MBB 105 DB	G-AZTI	SELF	P1	Truro - Redruth - Plymouth Apt - Truro			0.55								Sacral sore Alderson/ o'Byrne
Sep-05	MBB 105 DB	G-AZTI	SELF	P1	Truro - Plymouth FF - Airport			0.25								Brain Tumour Alderson/O'Byrne
Sep-05	MBB 105 DB	G-AZTI	SELF	P1	Airport - Bodmin - Bude - Plymouth FF - Truro			1.00								Fractured tib/fib Alderson/O'Byrne
Sep-05	MBB 105 DB	G-AZTI	Billings	P1	Truro - Bodmin A/F - Truro						1.15					Base Check O'Byrne
Sep-06	MBB 105 DB	G-AZTI	SELF	P1	Truro - Plymouth Apt - Truro			1.00								Burns Alderson/Williams
Sep-09	MBB 105 DB	G-AZTI	SELF	P1	Truro - Crafthole - Plymouth FF - St Austell - Truro			0.50								Miocardial Infarction Alderson/Williams
Sep-09	MBB 105 DB	G-AZTI	SELF	P1	Truro - Michelstowe - Bodmin A/F - Truro			0.35								Non injury RTA Alderson/Williams
Sep-10	MBB 105 DB	G-AZTI	SELF	P1	Truro local			0.10								RTA/Aborted Alderson/Williams
Sep-10	MBB 105 DB	G-AZTI	SELF	P1	Truro - King Harry - Truro			0.10								Coronary Alderson/Williams
Sep-10	MBB 105 DB	G-AZTI	SELF	P1	Truro - Bodmin - Truro			0.20								RTA Alderson/Williams
Sep-16	MBB 105 DB	G-AZTI	SELF	P1	Truro - Ruan High Lanes - Truro			0.10								RTA Harris/Williams
Sep-17	MBB 105 DB	G-AZTI	SELF	P1	Truro - Lands End - Truro			0.30								Fractured femur Harris/Williams
Sep-17	MBB 105 DB	G-AZTI	SELF	P1	Truro Plymouth Ho - Truro			0.50								Cervical paralysis Dr. Timmins/Harris
Sep-18	MBB 105 DB	G-AZTI	SELF	P1	Truro - Grampound - Tregony - Truro			0.15								Fractured clavical Dr Timmins/Harris
Sep-18	MBB 105 DB	G-AZTI	SELF	P1	Truro - Bude - Plymouth Apt			0.40								Renal Cholic Dr. Timmins/Harris

Year 1987 Month/Date	AIRCRAFT Type	Registration	Commander	Holder's Operating Capacity	Journey or Nature of Flight From (Dep)	To (Arr) (Times)	Day Flying Pilot-in-Command	Co-Pilot (P2)	Dual	Night Flying Pilot-in-Command	Co-Pilot (P2)	Dual	Instrument Flying	Instructor	MISSION
					Totals carried forward		4179.15	1092.50	289.40	321.35	140.25	32.25	494.30	966.40	
Sep-18	MBB 105 DB	G-AZTI	SELF	P1	Plymouth - Truro		0.20							Dr Timmins/Harris	Quadroplegic
Sep-18	MBB 105 DB	G-AZTI	SELF	P1	Truro - Bude - Plymouth FF - Truro		1.15							Harris/Williams	Motor Neurone Disease
Sep-18	MBB 105 DB	G-AZTI	SELF	P1	Truro - Portreath - Truro		0.10							Harris/Williams	RTA
Sep-19	MBB 105 DB	G-AZTI	SELF	P1	Truro - Roche - Truro		0.10							Harris/Williams	RTA
Sep-19	MBB 105 DB	G-AZTI	SELF	P1	Weather recce		0.15							Harris/Williams	Weather Recce
Sep-20	MBB 105 DB	G-AZTI	SELF	P1	Truro - St Mary's - Truro		1.00							Harris/Westaway	Compound fracture tib/fib
Sep-23	MBB 105 DB	G-AZTI	SELF	P1	Truro - Tregadillet - Plymouth FF - Truro		0.55							Harris/Westaway	Multiple injuries
Sep-23	MBB 105 DB	G-AZTI	SELF	P1	Truro - Zennor Head - Truro		0.20							Harris/Westaway	Fractured ankle
Sep-24	MBB 105 DB	G-AZTI	SELF	P1	Truro - Tintagel - Plymouth FF		0.30							Harris/Westaway	Asthma
Sep-24	MBB 105 DB	G-AZTI	SELF	P1	Plymouth FF - Looe - Plymouth FF - Apt		0.15							Harris/Westaway	Drowning (suicide?) Hypothermia
Sep-24	MBB 105 DB	G-AZTI	SELF	P1	Plymouth Apt - St Austell - Rock - Truro		0.30							Harris/Westaway	Carcenoma
Sep-25	MBB 105 DB	G-AZTI	SELF	P1	Truro - Plymouth FF - Truro		0.40							Harris/Westaway	Sub Arachnoid Haemorage
Sep-26	MBB 105 DB	G-AZTI	SELF	P1	truro - Bodmin		0.15							Harris/Westaway	Aborted
Sep-26	MBB 105 DB	G-AZTI	SELF	P1	Bodmin - Bodmin		0.30							Harris/Westaway	Aborted
Sep-26	MBB 105 DB	G-AZTI	SELF	P1	Bodmin - Roche - Truro		0.10							Harris Westaway	RTA
Sep-26	MBB 105 DB	G-AZTI	SELF	P1	Truro - St Teth - Truro		0.3							Harris/Westaway	Riding accident, Fractured Skull
Sep-26	MBB 105 DB	G-AZTI	SELF	P1	Truro - Gillan - Truro		0.25							Harris/Westaway	Crushed foot
Sep-26	MBB 105 DB	G-AZTI	SELF	P1	Truro - St Marys - Plymouth FF - Apt Truro		1.40							Harris/Westaway	Frctured Skull
Sep-27	MBB 105 DB	G-AZTI	SELF	P1	Truro - Port Isaac - Truro		0.25							Westaway/Slade	Peritonitis

Year 1987 Month/Date	AIRCRAFT Type	Registration	Commander	Holder's Operating Capacity	Journey or Nature of Flight From (Dep)	To (Arr) (Times)	Day Flying Pilot-in-Command	Co-Pilot (P2)	Dual	Night Flying Pilot-in-Command	Co-Pilot (P2)	Dual	Instrument Flying	Instructor	MISSION	
					Totals carried forward		4189.30	1092.50	289.40	321.35	140.25	32.25	494.30	966.40		
Sep-27	MBB 105 DB	G-AZTI	SELF	P1	Truro - Bude - Plymouth FF - Apt - Bodmin A/F		1.40								Fractured femur	Westaway/Slade
Sep-27	MBB 105 DB	G-AZTI	SELF	P1	Truro - Bodmin - Truro City		0.20								Head Injury	Westaway/Slade
Sep-27	MBB 105 DB	G-AZTI	SELF	P1	Truro City - Plymout Apt - Truro		0.20			0.20					Burn, scalds	Westaway + Dr ??
Sep-27	MBB 105 DB	G-AZTI	SELF	P1	Truro - Plymouth Apt - Truro					0.45					Hesd Injury	Westaway + Dr ??
Sep-30	MBB 105 DB	G-AZTI	SELF	P1	Truro - Tintagel - Truro		0.35								Burns to face	Westaway/Prissell
Sep-30	MBB 105 DB	G-AZTI	SELF	P1	Truro - Harlyn - Truro		0.20								Meningitis ??	Westaway/Prissell
Sep-30	MBB 105 DB	G-AZTI	SELF	P1	Truro - Bude - Plymouth FF - Apt - Bodmin A/F		0.45								Coronary	Westaway/Prissell
Sep-30	MBB 105 DB	G-AZTI	SELF	P1	Plymouth Apt - Plymouth FF - Truro		0.45								RTA	Westaway/Prissell
Oct-01	MBB 105 DB	G-AZTI	SELF	P1	Truro - Bodmin - Truro		0.20								Overdose	O'Byrne/Triggs
Oct-02	MBB 105 DB	G-AZTI	SELF	P1	Truro - Par - Plymouth FF		0.25								Fractured skull/hip/arm	Westaway/Triggs
Oct-02	MBB 105 DB	G-AZTI	SELF	P1	Plymouth FF - St Mellion - Plymouth FF Apt		0.20								Compound fracture femur/tib-fib	Westaway/Triggs
Oct-02	MBB 105 DB	G-AZTI	SELF	P1	Plymouth Apt - North Tamerton - Barnstable - Truro		1.15								Fractured femur	Westaway/Triggs
Oct-03	MBB 105 DB	G-AZTI	SELF	P1	Truro - St Agnes - Truro		0.20								Aid required	Westaway/Slade
Oct-04	MBB 105 DB	G-AZTI	SELF	P1	Truro - Plymouth Apt - Bodmin A/F		0.30								Sub Arachnoid	Harris/Slade
Oct-04	MBB 105 DB	G-AZTI	SELF	P1	Bodmin A/F - Bodmin - Truro		0.15								Overdose	Harris/Slade
Oct-04	MBB 105 DB	G-AZTI	SELF	P1	Truro - Plymouth FF - Truro		0.5								Sub Dural	Dr Morgan/Harris
Oct-04	MBB 105 DB	G-AZTI	SELF	P1	Truro - Lewennack - Plymouth FF - Truro		0.25								Aortic aneurism	Slade/Harris
Oct-08	MBB 105 DB	G-AZTI	SELF	P1	Truro - St Mawes - truro		0.10								Collapse	Harris/Slade
Oct-08	MBB 105 DB	G-AZTI	SELF	P1	Truro - Bodmin A/F		0.25								Listening watch	Harris/Slade

Year 1987 Month/Date	AIRCRAFT Type	Registration	Commander	Holder's Operating Capacity	Journey or Nature of Flight From (Dep)	To (Arr)	(Times)	Day Flying Pilot-in-Command	Co-Pilot (P2)	Dual	Night Flying Pilot-in-Comman	Co-Pilot (P2)	Dual	Instrument Flying	Instructor	MISSION
					Totals carried forward			4199.30	1092.50	289.40	323.05	140.25	32.25	494.30	966.40	
Oct-10	MBB 105 DB	G-AZTI	SELF	P1	Truro - Bodmin - Truro			0.20								RTA — Harris/Slade
Oct-10	MBB 105 DB	G-AZTI	SELF	P1	Truro St Just - Truro			0.30								Fractured leg — Harris/Slade
Oct-11	MBB 105 DB	G-AZTI	SELF	P1	Truro local			0.05								Testflight — Robinson/Nunn
Oct-11	MBB 105 DB	G-AZTI	SELF	P1	Truro - Looe - Plymouth FF			0.25								1. Fractured leg 2. Fractured wrist — Harris/Prissell
Oct-11	MBB 105 DB	G-AZTI	SELF	P1	Plymouth FF - Minions - Plymouth FF			0.10								Asthma attack — Harris/Prissell
Oct-11	MBB 105 DB	G-AZTI	SELF	P1	Plymouth FF - Apt - Truro - St Marys Truro			1.35								Fractured hip — Harris/Prissell
Oct-11	MBB 105 DB	G-AZTI	SELF	P1	Truro - Rock - Truro			0.20								Head and spinal injuries — Harris/Prissell
Oct-14	MBB 105 DB	G-AZTI	SELF	P1	Local Test flight post tail rotor change			0.10								Robinson
Oct-15	MBB 105 DB	G-AZTI	SELF	P1	Truro Test flight			0.05								Launder
Oct-15	MBB 105 DB	G-AZTI	SELF	P1	Truro - Bodmin - Truro			0.20								Throat cut — Harris/Prissell
Oct-16	MBB 105 DB	G-AZTI	SELF	P1	Truro test flight			0.05								Rhodes
Oct-16	MBB 105 DB	G-AZTI	SELF	P1	Truro - London Apprentice - Truro			0.15								Drunken Motorcyclist — Harris/Prissell
Oct-16	MBB 105 DB	G-AZTI	SELF	P1	Truro - The Lizard - Penzance - Truro			0.50								Myocardial Infarction — Harris/Prissell
Oct-17	MBB 105 DB	G-AZTI	SELF	P1	Truro Test Flight			0.05								Rhodes
Oct-21	MBB 105 DB	G-AZTI	SELF	P1	Truro local			0.05								
Oct-21	MBB 105 DB	G-AZTI	SELF	P1	Truro Penzance - St Marys			0.30								Terminal CA — Alderson + Dr ??
Oct-21	MBB 105 DB	G-AZTI	SELF	P1	St Marys - Penzance - Truro			0.20								Pulmonary embolism — Alderson/(Prissell)
Oct-21	MBB 105 DB	G-AZTI	SELF	P1	Truro - Ladock - Truro			0.10								Tractor accident — Alderson/Prsissell
Oct-22	MBB 105 DB	G-AZTI	SELF	P1	Truro - Penzance - Truro			0.25								Head Injury — Alderson/Prissell

Year 1987 Month/Date	AIRCRAFT Type	Registration	Commander	Holder's Operating Capacity	Journey or Nature of Flight From (Dep)	To (Arr)	Day Flying Pilot-in-Command	Co-Pilot (P2)	Dual	Night Flying Pilot-in-Command	Co-Pilot (P2)	Dual	Instrument Flying	Instructor	MISSION	
						Totals carried forward	4206.15	1092.50	289.40	323.05	140.25	32.25	494.30	966.40		
Oct-22	MBB 105 DB	G-AZTI	SELF	P1	Truro - Poole - Truro		0.10								Abdominal pains	Alderson/Prissell
Oct-22	MBB 105 DB	G-AZTI	SELF	P1	Truro - Boscastle - Truro		0.35								Overdose	Alderson/Prissell
Oct-23	MBB 105 DB	G-AZTI	SELF	P1	Truro - Penzance - Plymouth FF - Truro		1.05								Brain Tumour	Alderson + Dr ??
Oct-23	MBB 105 DB	G-AZTI	SELF	P1	Truro - Pentire Point - Truro		0.10								Fractured ankle	Alderson/Prissell
Oct-24	MBB 105 DB	G-AZTI	SELF	P1	Truro - St Merryn - Truro		0.20								Leg and chest injuries	Alderson/Prissell
Oct-24	MBB 105 DB	G-AZTI	SELF	P1	Truro - Wadebridge - Plymouth FF - Truro		0.45								Hotc pitch burns	Alderson/Prissell
Oct-25	MBB 105 DB	G-AZTI	SELF	P1	Truro - St Merryn - Bodmin A/F - Truro		0.35								Footballer (non injury)	Alderson/Prissell
Oct-28	MBB 105 DB	G-AZTI	SELF	P1	Truro local		0.05								Chief Officer (Len Holden) (Times)	Nick Rogers
Oct-28	MBB 105 DB	G-AZTI	SELF	P1	Truro - St Ives - Truro		0.20								Fractured ankle	Westaway/Triggs
Oct-28	MBB 105 DB	G-AZTI	SELF	P1	Truro - Tregony - Truro		0.10								EP/RTA Schizophrenic	Westaway/Triggs
Oct-29	MBB 105 DB	G-AZTI	SELF	P1	Truro - Davidstowe - St Mellion - Plymouth FF - Apt - Truro		0.55			0.20					1. Spinal injury 2. Collapse	Westaway/Triggs
Oct-29	MBB 105 DB	G-AZTI	SELF	P1	Truro - Tintagel - Plymouth Apt - Truro		0.35								Medical	Westaway/Triggs
Oct-30	MBB 105 DB	G-AZTI	SELF	P1	Truro - Bodmin A/F - Truro		0.35								s/by +Ian (Observer mag)	Westaway/Triggs
Oct-31	MBB 105 DB	G-AZTI	SELF	P1	Truro local		0.10								Dr Freeman and Paul Westaway	
Nov-01	MBB 105 DB	G-AZTI	SELF	P1	Truro local		0.05								Test Flight	Charlie/Ian Yeomans
Nov-01	MBB 105 DB	G-AZTI	SELF	P1	Truro - Roche - Truro City - CSSD		0.25								Fractured leg and arm	Harris/triggs/Yeomans
Nov-01	MBB 105 DB	G-AZTI	SELF	P1	Truro - Wadebridge - Truro		0.20								1. Fractured pelvis and arm 2. Glass in throat	Harris/Triggs/Yeomans
Nov-01	MBB 105 DB	G-AZTI	SELF	P1	Truro - Launcesto - Plymouth FF		0.25								Pellet in eye	Harris/Triggs
Nov-01	MBB 105 DB	G-AZTI	SELF	P1	Plymouth FF - Week St Mary - Plymouth FF - Apt - Truro		1.05								Dislocated shoulder	Harris/Triggs

Year 1987 Month/Date	AIRCRAFT Type	Registration	Commander	Holder's Operating Capacity	Journey or Nature of Flight (From - To)	Day Flying Pilot-in-Command	Day Flying Co-Pilot (P2)	Day Dual	Night Flying Pilot-in-Command	Night Flying Co-Pilot (P2)	Night Dual	Instrument Flying	Instructor	MISSION
					Totals carried forward	4215.05	1092.50	289.40	323.25	140.25	32.25	494.30	966.40	
Nov-04	MBB 105 DB	G-AZTI	SELF	P1	Truro - Blissland - Truro	0.15								Peumonia Harris/Prissell
Nov-04	MBB 105 DB	G-AZTI	SELF	P1	Truro - Penzance - Truro				0.10					Spainal fracture Harris/Prissell
Nov-05	MBB 105 DB	G-AZTI	SELF	P1	Truro - Camelford - Truro	0.35								Myocardial Infarction Harris/Prissell
Nov-06	MBB 105 DB	G-AZTI	SELF	P1	Truro - Bodmin - Padstow - Truro	0.25								Overdose Harris/Prissell
Nov-06	MBB 105 DB	G-AZTI	SELF	P1	Truro - Davidstowe - Plymouth Apt				0.30					Cardiac Westaway/Harris
Nov-07	MBB 105 DB	G-AZTI	SELF	P1	Plymouth Apt - St Teath - Truro	0.30			0.30					Reposition Westaway/Harris
Nov-07	MBB 105 DB	G-AZTI	SELF	P1	Truro - Helston - Truro	0.10								Fractured leg Harris/Prissell
Nov-07	MBB 105 DB	G-AZTI	SELF	P1	Truro - Bude - Barnstable - Truro	0.40			0.35					Internal Haemorage Harris/Prissell
Nov-08	MBB 105 DB	G-AZTI	SELF	P1	Truro - The Lizard - Truro	0.20								Epistaxis Harris/O'Byrne
Nov-08	MBB 105 DB	G-AZTI	SELF	P1	Truro - Morgan Porth - Truro	0.15								Fractured foot Harris/O'Byrne
Nov-08	MBB 105 DB	G-AZTI	SELF	P1	Truro - Carbis Bay - Truro	0.15								Head injury Harris/Obyrne
Nov-11	MBB 105 DB	G-AZTI	SELF	P1	Truro - Puloe - Plymouth FF - Apt - Truro	0.55								Myocardial infarction Harris/O'Byrne
Nov-12	MBB 105 DB	G-AZTI	SELF	P1	Truro - Local	0.05								
Nov-12	MBB 105 DB	G-AZTI	SELF	P1	Truro - Newquay - Truro	0.10								Myocardial Infarction Harris/O'Byrne
Nov-12	MBB 105 DB	G-AZTI	SELF	P1	Truro - Launceston - Plymouth FF - Truro	0.55								E.P. Age 7 Harris/O'Byrne
Nov-13	MBB 105 DB	G-AZTI	SELF	P1	Truro local	0.05								
Nov-13	MBB 105 DB	G-AZTI	SELF	P1	Truro - Bude - Plymouth Apt - Bodmin A/F	0.50								Retention Harris/Obyrne
Nov-13	MBB 105 DB	G-AZTI	SELF	P1	Bodmin A/F - St Austell - Truro City - Treliske	0.15								Compound fracture tib/fib Harris/O'Byrne
Nov-13	MBB 105 DB	G-AZTI	SELF	P1	Truro - Gribben Head - Truro	0.10								Post appendectomy complications Harris/O'Byrne

Year 1987 Month/Date	AIRCRAFT Type	Registration	Commander	Holder's Operating Capacity	Journey or Nature of Flight From (Dep)	To (Arr) (Times)	Pilot-in-Command	Day Flying Co-Pilot (P2)	Dual	Night Flying Pilot-in-Command	Co-Pilot (P2)	Dual	Instrument Flying	Instructor	MISSION
					Totals carried forward		4221.55	1092.50	289.40	325.05	140.25	32.25	494.30	966.40	
Nov-14	MBB 105 DB	G-AZTI	SELF	P1	Truro local		0.05								famil
Nov-14	MBB 105 DB	G-AZTI	SELF	P1	Truro - Gwithian - Truro city - CSSD		0.20								Compound fracture tib/fib · Harris/O'Byrne
Nov-14	MBB 105 DB	G-AZTI	SELF	P1	Truro - Penryn		0.05								Aborted · Harris/O'Byrne
Nov-14	MBB 105 DB	G-AZTI	SELF	P1	Penryn - Stithians - Truro		0.15								Fractured femur · Harris/O'Byrne
Nov-15	MBB 105 DB	G-AZTI	SELF	P1	Truro - Plymouth Truro		1.00								Spinal injury · Alderson/O'Byrne
Nov-18	MBB 105 DB	G-AZTI	SELF	P1	Truro local		0.05								famil
Nov-18	MBB 105 DB	G-AZTI	SELF	P1	Truro - Penzance - Plymouth Apt Castle Air - Truro		1.05								Brain tumour · Alderson/O'Byrne
Nov-18	MBB 105 DB	G-AZTI	SELF	P1	Truro - Cothele - Plymouth FF - Plymouth Apt - Truro		0.25			0.40					Fracture Pelvis · Alderson/O'Byrne
Nov-19	MBB 105 DB	G-AZTI	SELF	P1	Truro - Plymouth FF		0.20								Cerebral infarction · Alderson/O'Byrne
Nov-19	MBB 105 DB	G-AZTI	SELF	P1	Plymouth FF - Truro		0.30								Cerebral infarction · Alderson/O'Byrne
Nov-20	MBB 105 DB	G-AZTI	SELF	P1	Truro - Davidstowe Moor - Plymouth Apt - Bodmin A/F		0.50								CVA · Alderson/O'Byrne
Nov-20	MBB 105 DB	G-AZTI	SELF	P1	Bodmin A/F - Padstow - Truro		0.15								Convulsions · Alderson/O'Byrne
Nov-21	MBB 105 DB	G-AZTI	SELF	P1	Truro - Wadebridge - Truro		0.15								Partially severed finger · Alderson/O'Byrne
Nov-22	MBB 105 DB	G-AZTI	SELF	P1	Truro - Wadebridge - Truro		0.25								Gashed Kneecap · Alderson/Prissell
Nov-25	MBB 105 DB	G-AZTI	SELF	P1	Truro - Penzance - Plymouth Apt		1.00								Cancer - Chip light · Alderson/Prissell
Nov-25	MBB 105 DB	G-AZTI	SELF	P1	Plymouth Apt - Bude - Plymouth FF - Truro		0.35			0.20					Fractured Pelvis · Alderson/Prissell
Nov-28	MBB 105 DB	G-AZTI	SELF	P1	Truro - Goonhilly - Truro		0.20								Collapse · Alderson/Prissell
Nov-28	MBB 105 DB	G-AZTI	SELF	P1	Truro - Penrose - Truro		0.20								Acute retention · Alderson/Prissell
Nov-30	MBB 105 DB	G-AZTI	SELF	P1	Truro - Lanner - Truro - + local test flight		0.15								Suicide · Harris/Prissell

Year 1987 Month/Date	AIRCRAFT Type	Registration	Commander	Holder's Operating Capacity	Journey or Nature of Flight From (Dep) (Times) To (Arr)	Day Flying Pilot-in-Command	Co-Pilot (P2)	Dual	Night Flying Pilot-in-Command	Co-Pilot (P2)	Dual	Instrument Flying	Instructor	MISSION
					Totals carried forward	4230.20	1092.50	289.40	326.05	140.25	32.25	494.30	966.40	
Dec-01	MBB 105 DB	G-AZTI	SELF	P1	Truro - Launceston - Plymouth FF - Apt	0.35								1. Head & chest 2. Chest and Back Harris/Prissell
Dec-01	MBB 105 DB	G-AZTI	SELF	P1	Apt - Launceston, Red Post - Barnstable - Truro	1.00								Severe retention Harris/Prissell
Dec-02	MBB 105 DB	G-AZTI	SELF	P1	Truro - Four Lanes - Truro	0.05			0.10					Head injury Harris/Prissell
Dec-03	MBB 105 DB	G-AZTI	SELF	P1	Truro local	0.05								test flight
Dec-03	MBB 105 DB	G-AZTI	SELF	P1	Truro - Boscastle - Truro	0.35								Fractured tib/fib Harris/Prissell
Dec-03	MBB 105 DB	G-AZTI	SELF	P1	Truro - Launceston - Plymouth Apt - St Austell - Truro	1.00								C.A. Harris/Prissell
Dec-04	MBB 105 DB	G-AZTI	SELF	P1	Truro - Mabe - Plymouth Apt - Truro	1.20								Renal Dr Simcox/Harris
Dec-07	MBB 105 DB	G-AZTI	SELF	P1	Truro - Tintagel - Plymouth Apt - Truro	0.55								Angina Harris/Williams
Dec-09	MBB 105 DB	G-AZTI	SELF	P1	Truro - Clawton - Plymouth FF - Apt	0.40								1. Head injury 2. Spinal injury RTA Harris/Williams
Dec-09	MBB 105 DB	G-AZTI	SELF	P1	Apt - Clawton - St Merryn - Truro	0.35								Post viral infection Harris/Williams
Dec-09	MBB 105 DB	G-AZTI	SELF	P1	Truro - Nanpean - Truro	0.10								E.P Fit Harris/Williams
Dec-10	MBB 105 DB	G-AZTI	SELF	P1	Truro - Bude - Plymouth Apt	0.40								1. Perforated ulcer 2. Retention Harris/Williams
Dec-10	MBB 105 DB	G-AZTI	SELF	P1	Apt - Bude - Plymouth FF	0.35								Fractured ankle Harris/Williams
Dec-10	MBB 105 DB	G-AZTI	SELF	P1	Plymouth FF - Launceston - Plymouth FF - Apt	0.30								Haemetemesis Harris/Williams
Dec-10	MBB 105 DB	G-AZTI	SELF	P1	Plymouth Apt - Lanhydrock - Truro	0.15								Haemetemesis Harris/Williams
Dec-11	MBB 105 DB	G-AZTI	SELF	P1	Truro - Bodmin A/F - Bodmin - Truro	0.30								Gall Stanes Harris/Williams
Dec-11	MBB 105 DB	G-AZTI	SELF	P1	Truro -Camelford - Plymouth FF - Truro	1.05								Deep vein thrombosis Harris/Williams
Dec-15	MBB 105 DB	G-AZTI	SELF	P1	Truro local	0.05								Test flight
Dec-16	MBB 105 DB	G-AZTI	SELF	P1	Truro - Bude - Barstable - Truro	1.35								Abdominal pains Harris/Williams

Year 1987 Month/Date	AIRCRAFT Type	Registration	Commander	Holder's Operating Capacity	Journey or Nature of Flight From (Dep)	To (Arr) [Times]	Day Flying Pilot-in-Command	Co-Pilot (P2)	Dual	Night Flying Pilot-in-Command	Co-Pilot (P2)	Dual	Instrument Flying	Instructor	MISSION
					Totals carried forward		4242.35	1092.50	289.40	326.15	140.25	32.25	494.30	966.40	
Dec-18	MBB 105 DB	G-AZTI	SELF	P1	Truro - St Austell - Truro		0.20								Asthma Emphasema Westaway/Williams
Dec-18	MBB 105 DB	G-AZTI	SELF	P1	Truro - Mullion - Truro		0.20								Laryngal spasms Westaway/Williams
Dec-18	MBB 105 DB	G-AZTI	SELF	P1	Truro - Mullion - Truro		0.10								Muscular weakness Westaway/Williams
Dec-22	MBB 105 DB	G-AZTI	SELF	P1	Truro - Padstow - Truro		0.25								Appendicitis Westaway/O'Byrne
Dec-23	MBB 105 DB	G-AZTI	SELF	P1	Truro - Indian Queens - City - CSSD		0.25								Head, chest, and leg injuries Westaway/Slade
Dec-24	MBB 105 DB	G-AZTI	SELF	P1	Truro - Bodmin A/F - Bodmin Moor - Truro		0.45								Attempted suicide Wesataway/Slade
Dec-29	MBB 105 DB	G-AZTI	SELF	P1	Truro local		0.05								Test flight
Dec-30	MBB 105 DB	G-AZTI	SELF	P1	Truro - Daymer Bay - Truro		0.25								Fractured leg Westaway/Williams
Dec-31	MBB 105 DB	G-AZTI	SELF	P1	Truro - Bude - Plymouth Apt		0.35								Abdominal pains Westaway/Williams
Dec-31	MBB 105 DB	G-AZTI	SELF	P1	Apt - Boscastle - Plymouth FF - Truro		1.05								Pulmonary embolysm Westaway/Williams
Jan-05	MBB 105 DB	G-AZTI	SELF	P1	Truro - Davidstowe - Plymouth FF - Bodmin A/F - Truro		0.55								Eye injury Alderson/Slade
Jan-07	MBB 105 DB	G-AZTI	SELF	P1	Truro - Penzance - Truro		0.25								Fractured arm Alderson/Slade
Jan-07	MBB 105 DB	G-AZTI	SELF	P1	Truro (PR flight) local		0.05								PR Flight +1 Alderson/Slade
Jan-11	MBB 105 DB	G-AZTI	SELF	P1	Truro Bodmin A/F		0.10								On standby
Jan-11	MBB 105 DB	G-AZTI	SELF	P1	Bodmin A/F - Delabole - Truro		0.20								Asthma Harris/Williams
Jan-11	MBB 105 DB	G-AZTI	SELF	P1	Truro - Launceston - Plymouth FF - Apt		0.3								RTA, fractured femur Harris/Williams
Jan-11	MBB 105 DB	G-AZTI	SELF	P1	Apt - Camelford - Plymouth FF - Truro		0.45								Stroke Harris/Williams
Jan-12	MBB 105 DB	G-AZTI	SELF	P1	Truro - Lewennack - Plymouth Apt		0.30								Spinal Harris/Williams
Jan-12	MBB 105 DB	G-AZTI	SELF	P1	Apt - Penzance - Truro		0.55								Fractured femur Harris/Williams

Year 1987 Month/Date	AIRCRAFT Type	Registration	Commander	Holder's Operating Capacity	Journey or Nature of Flight From (Dep)	To (Arr)	Day Flying Pilot-in-Command	Co-Pilot (P2)	Dual	Night Flying Pilot-in-Comman	Co-Pilot (P2)	Dual	Instru-ment Flying	Instructor	MISSION	
					Totals carried forward		4252.45	1092.50	289.40	326.15	140.25	32.25	494.30	966.40		
Jan-13	MBB 105 DB	G-AZTI	SELF	P1	Truro - Budock - Truro		0.10								Testiculitis	Harris/Williams
Jan-13	MBB 105 DB	G-AZTI	SELF	P1	Truro - Bodmin - Truro		0.20								Adison's Disease	Harris/Williams
Jan-14	MBB 105 DB	G-AZTI	SELF	P1	Truro - Constantine - Truro		0.10								Head Injury	Harris/Williams
Jan-14	MBB 105 DB	G-AZTI	SELF	P1	Truro - Polperro - Truro		0.25								Coronary (deceased)	Harris Williams
Jan-15	MBB 105 DB	G-AZTI	SELF	P1	Truro - Zelah - Truro		0.10								Cut fingers, no transport	Harris/Williams
Jan-15	MBB 105 DB	G-AZTI	SELF	P1	Truro - Penzance - Truro		0.20								Pneumothorax	Harris/Williams

ABOUT THE AUTHOR

The author lives in Cornwall and has based the Jack Mawgan novels in and around the South West of England. He is an ex-Navy helicopter pilot who for almost fifty years has worked as a pilot, instructor and consultant in diverse and fascinating locations around the world. From Greenland to The Falkland Islands, the Russian Taiga to the African bush, Brazil to the North Sea. He has flown Air Ambulances, Police and Search and Rescue helicopters so knows a thing or two about how they help to save lives. His successful 'Jack Mawgan Trilogy' now has a fourth book to add to the tales of Cornwall's most successful and irrepressible homicide detective.

-------- 0 -------

The Jack Mawgan Trilogy Book 1
FOR THE PRICE OF A HAT

Jack Mawgan was a highly successful homicide detective until fate dealt him a tragic blow. Walking away from his career in the Police Force he is persuaded to take up a new career in one of the other emergency services by his GP wife, Pamela. He joins the Ambulance Service to become a paramedic, but his instincts for solving violent crime prove impossible to leave behind. In his first case in this new role, a millionaire businessman from Glasgow is assassinated at his home in Cornwall. Jack attends the scene of the murder and soon becomes embroiled in chasing down the murderer. The killer's trail leads to an aristocratic crook and his henchman who both have much blood on their hands after more than a decade of crime and corruption. The situation rapidly deteriorates and leads to life-threatening consequences for him, his family and his friends that are only resolved after more murder and mayhem.

The Jack Mawgan Trilogy Book 2
RENDER UNTO CAESAR

After years of training, Jack Mawgan is about to fulfil his ambition to become a qualified paramedic when an incident involving a young Muslim found naked on a Cornish road in broad daylight draws him into the sinister world of 'Extraordinary Rendition'. This campaign was run by the US security services and involved their operatives in torture in their search for information about Al Qaeda's activities. Jack's involvement sets off a chain of events that leads him to the depths of the African interior in pursuit of a self-proclaimed jihadist fomenting rebellion and heavily involved in the drugs trade.

The Jack Mawgan Trilogy Book 3
THE MARK

To suggest that those generous souls who put themselves forward as trustees of the many Air Ambulance Trusts around the country are uniformly evil is, of course, hyperbole. I am sure they are entirely without blemish, but unfortunately, if that were true it would not provide an interesting plot for my story, so I beg them not to take my aspersions seriously. That said we know from our newspapers that corruption is everywhere and our public services are particularly vulnerable to the few who break our bond of trust. Occasionally it is our elected politicians that let us down. Lord Acton, a prominent historian of the Victorian era, once said in a letter to Mary Gladstone (daughter of the Prime Minister, William Gladstone, and his confidante and advisor).

"I cannot accept your canon that we are to judge Pope and King, unlike other men, with a favourable presumption that they did no wrong. If there is any presumption, it is the other way against holders of power, increasing as the power increases. Historic responsibility has to make up for the want of legal responsibility. Power tends to corrupt, and absolute power corrupts absolutely. Great men are almost always bad men, even when they exercise influence and not authority: still more when you add the tendency or the certainty of corruption by authority. There is no worse heresy than that the office sanctifies the holder of it." (Wikipedia)

Whether you agree with Lord Acton or not we must always be prepared to take our leaders to task when they overstep the mark. This book tells a tale that would make Lord Acton shake his head at the way our modern society is developing.

The latest Jack Mawgan thriller

THE ONE ROMANIAN

"Another tightly written thriller to supplement the highly successful Jack Mawgan Trilogy. This time Jack takes on a dark and callous foe whose evil methods include medieval torture delivered under a cloak of religious fanaticism."

A knock on the door of his London apartment – a beautiful woman needs his help. Jack sets out on another crime-fighting adventure that nearly costs him his life.

Once again Jack finds he is unable to resist the challenge to his detective skills. He is faced with the apparently motiveless murder of four Romanian men who are found floating in the River Thames.

What could possible link the murders in London to Rome, Bucharest and The Falklands? The answer involves shocking revelations of a British plan to launch a nuclear attack in South America and uncovers corruptions in the Catholic Church on a global scale.

Jack has his work cut out.